THE INTELLECTUAL
BASE OF
SOCIAL WORK PRACTICE

Social Work Education and Practice:
A Saul Horowitz Jr. Memorial Series
of the Hunter College School of Social Work

These contributions to the study of social work — written by faculty, students, and graduates of the Hunter College School of Social Work — are published in honor of a distinguished community leader, Saul Horowitz Jr. (1925–1975)

Social Work in Health Services: An Academic Practice Partnership

edited by Phillis Caroff and Mildred Mailick   1980

The Intellectual Base of Social Work Practice: Tools for Thought in a Helping Profession

Harold Lewis   1982

THE INTELLECTUAL BASE OF SOCIAL WORK PRACTICE

Tools for Thought in a Helping Profession

»»   ««

HAROLD LEWIS

Dean
Hunter College School of Social Work

THE LOIS AND SAMUEL SILBERMAN FUND
THE HAWORTH PRESS
New York   *1982*

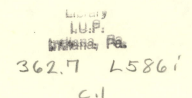
Library of Congress Cataloging in Publication Data

Lewis, Harold.
   The intellectual base of social work practice.

   (Saul Horowitz Jr. memorial series)
   Includes bibliographical references and index.
   1. Social work education. 2. Social service.
I. Title. II. Series.
HV10.5.L48   361.3   82–5593
ISBN 0–86656–176–5   AACR2

The Intellectual Base of Social Work Practice: Tools for Thought in a Helping Profession is copublished by The Lois and Samuel Silberman Fund, Inc., 133 East 79 Street, New York, New York 10021, and by The Haworth Press, Inc., 28 East 22 Street, New York, New York 10010

Designed and produced by
THE BOOKMAKERS, INCORPORATED
Editorial, Design, Graphic, and Production Services to the Publishing Industry
Case of the Hunter College School of Social Work
Anniversary Edition designed by Joseph Caroff

Manufactured in the United States of America

TO CELIA, AMY, AND BETH

Contents

Foreword   *ix*

Preface   *xi*

Acknowledgments   *xiii*

Introduction   Learning to Help People   *3*

PART I   THE NATURE OF WORK,
THE WORKER, THE RECIPIENT,
AND THE PRODUCT

One   The Nature of Work   *9*

Two   The Worker, the Recipient, and the
Product   *17*

PART II   THE ELEMENTS OF SKILL

Three   Intellectual Tools   *41*

Four   Theory   *61*

Five   Ethics   *83*

Six   Knowledge   *105*

Seven   Values   *127*

Eight   Style   *147*

Nine   Skill   *161*

PART III   WORK AS ACTION

Ten   Understanding the Elements of Work   *177*

Eleven   Interventions, Assessment, Outcome,
and an Approach to Practice   *189*

Twelve   Reasoning in Practice   *223*

Thirteen   Context   *251*

Index   *254*

»»   ««

Foreword

THE INTELLECTUAL BASE OF SOCIAL WORK PRACTICE: Tools for Thought in a Helping Profession, by Harold Lewis, is the second volume of the Saul Horowitz Jr. Memorial Series of the Hunter College School of Social Work. The series was established by The Lois and Samuel Silberman Fund to honor a distinguished community leader, the late Saul Horowitz Jr., by promoting the publication of scholarly work in the field of social work by faculty, students, and graduates of the School.

It is particularly fitting this year that the Publications Committee should select the work of Dr. Lewis to coincide with the twenty-fifth anniversary celebration of the Hunter College School of Social Work. Dean Lewis has provided outstanding leadership in the School, in the University, in the community, and in the profession. His efforts have contributed significantly to the School's recognition as a leading institution in graduate social work education. His scholarly work reflects a level of intellectual excellence in which those of us in the profession share great pride. We believe that this work makes a significant contribution not only to social work but also to the larger arena of the human service professions.

Phyllis Caroff, *Chairperson*
Saul Horowitz Jr.
Publications Committee

»» ««

Preface

A YEAR SPENT at the Center for Advanced Study in the Behavioral Sciences pursuing an interest in how the brain knows it is being asked a question stimulated the essays that make up this volume. This interest in turn originated in another concern—a desire to improve education for professional practice. It occured to me that the manner in which information was organized and processed for storage in memory and then recovered for action was intimately connected with the inner-directed questions practitioners put to themselves when rendering their services.[1]

Such inner-directed questions signal the brain to prepare to respond to what is being stored. In common with all questions, they alert the brain to prepare to do more than store what is being communicated to it. But inner-directed questions of practitioners seek guidance from the brain for critical judgments that must be both appropriate and timely. The practitioner must take prompt action, lest opportunities for intervention be lost as well. In this respect, they differ from the ordinary.

My educational interest in this subject stemmed from the belief that the inner-directed question would serve its function more efficiently if it were properly designed—if it identified, packaged, and processed the essentials of what is to be communicated in a manner appropriate for quick recognition and recovery in practice situations.[2] Whereas theory and its

1. For a definition of *recovery* as used in this book, see p. 12.
2. Donald A. Norman, *Memory and Attention* (New York: John Wiley & Sons, 1969).

derived propositions effectively achieve such efficiency in the disciplines, professional interventions also require principles and rules that are specific to their time and place and applicable to particular cases. Together, they inform both practitioners' actions and their inner-directed inquiries.

I did not expect my question to be answered during my stay at the Center, and in this I was not disappointed; but my pursuit did clarify less difficult and more immediately useful issues confronting teachers who seek to educate practitioners for a professional practice.

In the essays that make up this volume, I have concentrated on one profession—social work—though the approach taken and introductory analysis attempted would, I believe, be equally useful for teachers in other professions. In sharing the results of my inquiry with my readers, I hope that they find merit in the subjects considered and that some may be motivated to persue them further, while avoiding the pitfalls they identify in my work. Were this to occur, the time and thought devoted to the preparation of these essays will have been more than justified.

»» ««

Acknowledgments

MY YEAR at the Center for Advanced Study in the Behavioral Sciences provided the ideal environment in which to initiate this inquiry. Herbert Aptekar and Ruth Smalley gave generously of their time in reacting critically to various sections of the work in progress. Nine successive classes of doctoral students, for whom much of the content served as course text, contributed to clarification and deeper appreciation of the complexity of the subject, the difficulty of communicating its content, and the introductory nature of the discussion offered here. Colleagues who have had access to earlier drafts were generous in their responses. Florence Vigilante deserves a special expression of appreciation for her persistence in encouraging me to revise an earlier version. The product, while owing much to these supports, remains in its shortcomings the authors alone. Joe Caroff's design of the cover for the special Hunter College School of Social Work twenty-fifth anniversary edition contributed his remarkable talent to the reader's first eye-contact with this volume for a most pleasing result.

THE INTELLECTUAL
BASE OF
SOCIAL WORK PRACTICE

»» ««

Learning to Help People

MY FRIEND BOB went through graduate school during the Depression, earning a master's degree in history in 1933. Before the Second World War, he worked as a historian on a dance project sponsored by the WPA. Later he took a job as a social investigator with the department of welfare, which he left to serve in the armed services. In 1946, when he was honorably discharged with the rank of captain, he decided to go back to school for a second master's, this one in social work.

Bob attended the New York School of Social Work, which at that time was located in the old Russell Sage Building, on Twenty-second Street and Lexington Avenue in Manhattan. One day Bob was standing near the public phones in the lobby with a crowd of fellow students when a truck pulled up in front of the building and its driver came in to use a phone. When he finished his call, he tapped Bob on the shoulder and asked, "What goes on here? Why all these people?"

Bob explained, "This is a school."

The driver asked, "What do they study here?"

After thinking a bit, Bob hesitantly answered, "They learn how to help people."

The driver stared at him in surprise and exclaimed, "For that you have to go to school?"

Although the driver's question amused Bob, it nagged at

him as well; and he still remembered the incident many years later when we both taught in a graduate school of social work. Despite evidence to the contrary, many people in all walks of life believe that if you want to help people, good intentions and common sense are enough. They wonder why formal training is necessary.

If Bob had pressed the trucker to explain why he wondered about schooling for those who want to help others, the driver's explanation might have provided his personal slant on what he considered obvious. If the trucker were a college graduate — or possibly a drop-out from graduate education — his explanation might have echoed the opinion of many educators in the social and behavioral sciences, who see such helpers as social workers as *doers*. In their view, the helping professional simply translates social and behavioral science into action. Thus they see the social worker primarily as a feeling person, not as a knowledgeable professional.[1] They regard the skill of the helper as a technical achievement that consists in the art of applying specific techniques to particular situations. In fact, they might even insist that of the three attributes — knowledge, value, and action — only the third is so unique to social work that it alone should be judged in evaluating professional practice. Like the truck driver, they could ask: Why an advanced graduate degree when all that needs to be learned is best mastered in the doing? Why not rely on an apprenticeship (with occasional inputs of the knowledge that the social and behavioral sciences produce) for the proper preparation of the helper?

My friend Bob is an intellectual, however, and his chosen profession — social work — consists largely of mental work. This profession attracts persons primarily interested in mental work, in contrast to manual work. That the profession

1. Margaret Blenkner, "Obstacles to Evaluative Research in Casework," *Social Casework* 31 (February-March 1950): 97–105.

also attracts persons whose talents for relating to people may be above average, is an added advantage. It is not a substitute for the intellectual interest that prompts an individual to pursue a specialized advanced education. This book therefore focuses on the intellectual element in social work practice. It is an answer, in part, to the truck driver's question.

A good question signals what is acceptable as an answer.[2] "For *that* [helping people] you have to go to school?" is such a question. It asks for a response that indicates some of the intellectual work to be mastered through formal education. The sequence of chapters in this book has been ordered accordingly: Part I describes the nature of the work, of the worker, of the recipient, and of the product; Part II surveys what is involved in the development of skill in practice; and Part III elaborates on the intellectual work to be mastered in applying this skill. Finally, the conclusion recognizes the limits of the analysis and attempts to locate the social worker as such in the wider societal context in which practice takes place.

2. Felix S. Cohen, "What is a Question?" *The Monist* 34 (1929): 350–64; Paul Edwards, "Why?" in *Encyclopedia of Philosophy* ed. Paul Edwards (New York: Macmillan Co., 1967), 8: 296–302; Charles Hamblin, "Questions," ibid., 7: 49–51; David Harrah, "A Logic of Questions and Answers," *Philosophy of Science* 28 (January 1961): 40–46; R. M. MacIver, "The Modes of the Question Why," *Journal of Social Philosophy* 5 (October 1939–July 1940): 197–205; John M. D. Wheatley, "Deliberative Questions," *Analysis* 15, no. 3 (January 1955): 49–60.

»» ««

PART I

The Nature of Work,
the Worker, the Recipient,
and the Product

CHAPTER ONE

>» «<

The Nature of Work

INTELLECTUAL WORK shares many attributes with manual work, but this relationship may not be immediately obvious or easy to explain. My father, a sewing machine operator for close to fifty years, first made me aware of this problem when he sought to understand exactly what I did to earn a living. When I said that I was a social worker, he usually nodded, raised one eyebrow quizzically, and asked, "So what do you do?" Since I was employed in research work, I would talk about the studies I was doing. He would listen and voice appreciation for the good that might come from my effort. Inevitably, he would end our exchange with the same question, "But what is the *work* you do?" In frustration, I concluded that a prerequisite for answering his question was some clarification of the concept of *work*.

Work

All work can be divided into three parts.[1] First, for there to be a call to do any work, there must be a *condition to be*

1. Paul Schrecker, *Work and History: An Essay on the Structure of Civilization* (New York: Thomas Y. Crowell Co., 1971), pp. 12–18. The definition of work developed by Professor Schrecker in this study of civilization underpins the paradigm used in this analysis. When the literature of social work describes practice, it is of course describing the work done by social workers. In addition, the literature describing the profession from sociological, psychological, economic, and political

altered.[2] For people who prefer things as they are, work intended to change conditions is to be avoided. Others may perceive conditions they would like to alter but feel that the cost in effort required to bring about the desired change is more than they are willing to invest. For either of these persons, there is no call for work. Of course, for those lazy few, for whom even a minimal exertion is too much, avoidance is not a preference but a disorder; and as such it falls outside the scope of this analysis.

In addition to a condition to be altered, there must also be an *investment of effort* for work to occur. The condition can be altered only by an investment of effort on the part of the worker. But because a social worker uses the mind rather than the hand and because it is often difficult to identify and describe mental effort, the nature and scope of much of social work remains obscure.

The third element of work is less tangible than either the condition to be altered or the effort to be expended. It is the *worker's necessary belief* that a condition can be improved through efforts made to change it. In the absence of a belief, there is no rational purpose in the expenditure of resources to bring about a change.

These three elements are essential for any work—intellectual or manual—to be done. Where one or more is lacking, change may occur, but work is not being done.

---

perspectives also focuses on the work done by social workers. Although Schrecker's concept is abstract, it can also be generalized to all of human work in a historical and cross-cultural perspective that is particularly appropriate for the analysis attempted in this chapter.

2. Herbert Aptekar asks "May I dare to raise a question whether social work is inherently directed to change? It certainly has come to be equated with change in our American minds. . . . We in the West (and a lot of people in the East today who have become 'Westernized') do want to master and change society and social relations. But that does not mean that there can't be social work which is not directed to change [maintenance of a desirable status quo]." Personal communication, 14 October 1970.

Thus it is possible to believe that a condition can be improved but do nothing to achieve it. To recognize how prevalent this possibility is, one needs only to recall all the studies that demonstrate either the inadequacies of available housing for poor families, or the lack of health care for the medically indigent, or the restrictions on educational opportunities for the financially disadvantaged and then to list all the suggested improvements that have not been made. It is also possible to expend considerable effort unintentionally altering a condition once thought ideal. When Linus Pauling warned about the effects of radioactive fallout from atomic testing, he was pointing out an unintended by-product of otherwise intended effort. The healthy atmosphere was contaminated; and although a condition was changed, improvement was not the result. Finally, as the expression "to knock one's head against a stone wall" suggests, misdirected effort is not likely to achieve much improvement in a condition one wants to change.

>>   <<

It would be gratifying if I could conclude my analysis of work with this description of its three elements. But an additional factor intervenes: For work to occur, these elements must all be present concurrently; and when all are present, complications develop in their interaction. These complications in turn require that the worker be capable of judgments at once more difficult and more informed.

Thus, when a condition to be altered is viewed in relation to a goal to be achieved, an unmet need must be specified and purpose and objectives must be considered. For example, we can believe in the possibility of reducing the number of unwanted pregnancies among unmarried girls in their early teens without being clear as to the nature of the unmet need we should meet to achieve this objective. Should we cultivate a puritanical view of premarital sexual activity?

KEY TERMS

Several relatively common English words are used throughout this book in a specific technical sense. Although this special terminology should be clear from the context, the following brief glossary provides concise definitions.

VALUES. Those enduring beliefs we hold about what is to be preferred as good and right in our conduct and in our existence as human beings.

ETHICS. Those rules of conduct that direct us to act in a manner consistant with the values we profess. ETHICAL IMPERATIVES are therefore the rules of conduct to be preferred.

COMMENDATIONS. The *shoulds, oughts, musts,* and *wills* that monitor possible deviations from ethical imperatives. They are intended to dispel any doubts that the prescribed action is also a desirable action.

PURPOSES. Those intentions set up as objects or ends to be attained. They include actions whose execution would further their realization.

GOALS. The conditions to be achieved as a result of effort expended. Such conditions are believed to represent the realization of preferred values.

OBJECTIVES. The outcomes of work that are directly related to effort expended. A range of objectives may collectively be viewed as contributory to the achievement of an ultimate goal.

NEED. A judgment that a condition that exists should be altered to achieve a preferred end and that expenditure of resource is warranted to make this change possible.

RECOVERY. The process whereby the practitioner takes from memory stored knowledge for use in practice. It is not to be confused with the process of identification and selection of information usually designated as *retrieval.* The former includes the latter, but it incorporates changes and transformations of stored materials by mental associations.

Should we provide widespread information about and access to contraceptive devices? Should we restrict the opportunities for the unsupervised mixing of the sexes in the early teens? Although the goal is accepted, no definition has been either proposed or universally accepted that specifies which need, if met, would achieve that objective. Nor have programs intended to educate teenagers in self-restraint reduced pregnancies — even when the youngsters showed they had the knowledge that education was intended to convey. In any work, it is far easier to designate a condition to be altered and a goal to be achieved than it is to specify the relevant unmet need and the objectives that need to be accomplished to assure that the goal will be met.

Certain attributes of work are so intimately linked to the consideration of goals in relation to the resources that must be expended to achieve them that they foster equally complex considerations. Goals reflect the ultimate values to which the worker appeals in justifying the effort expended to alter a condition. For example, if a child-welfare worker did not believe that loving and considerate care in a child's own family is normally preferable to institutional or other out-of-home care, there would be little justification for the effort expended to help children return to their homes. This relationship between goals and values invests programs of intervention with their ideological content, thereby complicating their design and sponsorship. Resources, in turn, are utilized through the application of methods that generate a helpful process. At this point, choices can become complicated. For example, the selection of individual, group, or family counseling as the best method for guiding the child and his or her family in the direction that will promote the child's return to his own home under acceptable conditions complicates the decision about allocation of resources.

Such complexities discourage a simplistic view of work. Other complexities evolve when the conditions to be altered

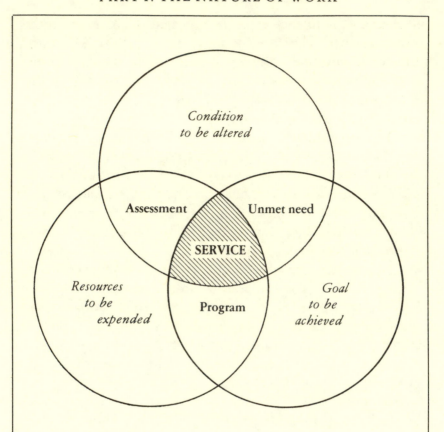

Figure 1. This figure suggests *(1)* that when an existing condition is judged to be subject to change through the expenditure of resources and a preferred end (goal) would be achieved as a result, the condition is endowed with the necessary attributes of an unmet need; *(2)* that when an end to be achieved justifies a claim on available resources, the form in which this claim is embodied is a program of action that incorporates the modes of intervention and the allocated resources into policies and procedures; and *(3)* that when an effort is made to determine the resources required to alter a condition in a preferred direction, the result is an assessment of the work to be done. See Chapter 10 for a more detailed analysis of the elements of figure 1.

are juxtaposed to the resources required to bring about the desired change. The mix here generates that most critical and difficult intellectual task in all mental work: accurate assessment of the nature of the need and of the appropriate action to meet it. The history of human service professions is replete with examples of the pitfalls that accompany efforts at assessment. Good diagnostic tools are the backbone of any profession's claim to competence; and many of the techniques of the professions represent the culmination of lengthy intellectual efforts—including trial and error, experiment and demonstration, discovery and invention. The intellectual task of carrying out a good assessment—describing a need and matching it to an appropriate intervention—is enormously complex. For this very reason, it is least appreciated by those who do not participate in its risks and challenges.

The relationships among the three elements of work and the complexities their interaction generates are shown in Figure 1.

ELEMENTS OF WORK

I HAVE NOT YET CONSIDERED what develops when all three elements are concurrently related to each other, which in fact is how they occur in practice. The result of their interaction is in fact more difficult to appreciate than anything thus far presented. Later, after we have considered the nature of skill in greater detail, we can spend some time on this aspect of work. For the present it suffices to give it a label and designate its unique character as used in this text.

What comes into being through the concurrent interaction of all three elements of work—although it is not present in any of these elements considered separately—is the possibility of *service*. Service, as I use the term, occurs when a recipient's need is met through the use of a resource provided by the worker's effort on the recipient's behalf.

Specialization

People tend to specialize in order to work more efficiently and effectively. With the passage of time, they are able to develop some expertise in implementing changes appropriate to their intentions. When the collective expertise of a group of people becomes recognized, sanctioned, and supported by society, that group's unique efforts are designated by a title. Depending on many attributes and circumstances, such titles include trades and professions. They share a common understanding of the condition that should be changed, of the goal to be achieved, and of the means for expending effort to bring about the desired change with more than usual efficiency and effectiveness. The specialized workers on whose work I concentrate in this study are a species called *social workers* within the genus *Professional*. Their peculiar attributes must be appreciated if the subsequent discussion of their intellectual work is to be properly understood.

CHAPTER TWO

»» ««

The Worker, the Recipient, and the Product

W<small>E USUALLY SEEK</small> professional help for ourselves because we need assistance in altering a condition we find troublesome. If we could achieve the same change without help, we would rarely want the guidance of an expert. In fact, whenever such guidance is provided in situations where we see no need for it and do not invite it, we regard it as an intrusion — a violation of our autonomy — and therefore something to be resisted. When we want and need help, however, selecting a professional helper can be a difficult task. If we have no choice — whether for financial, technical, organizational, or other reasons — we may have to accept help from a professional worker whose abilities we must presume to be adequate on the basis of credentials, sponsorship, or reputation.

Ideally, were we given a choice, what criteria would we use in selecting a helper? We would probably base our selection on one or more of the following: What the helper knows, what he or she can do, and what sort of person he or she is reputed to be. Consider these three attributes as they apply to the specialized professional practitioner called *social worker*.

What Must She Know?

The social worker seeks to influence not only human growth and behavior but also the social environment in which such growth and behavior occur. Hence, she must be informed about these elements. She should also be informed about the nature of services and the manner in which they are rendered. This presumes both a familiarity with the history of service and service organizations, and an understanding first of their structures and functions and second of the purposes for which they are appropriate. Most important, a social worker must have a practical grasp of the resources and techniques utilized in her work if she is to participate actively in practice and not merely passively observe it. Finally, she should be able to recognize success or failure in her efforts, be able to evaluate the consequences of either, and know how to analyze and improve her practice as a result. If we could be assured that our potential helper was knowledgeable in all these areas, we would certainly be more inclined to seek her services.

What Can She Do?

There is, of course, much room for a gap between knowing and doing — between theory and practice. Each of us can draw from personal experience and history situations when knowing what to do in a situation provided no assurance, even given both opportunity and motivation, of the ability to do it. Knowing *what* and *why* is an essential prerequisite to appropriate action, since such knowledge tells us where to look and what to look for.[1] Such knowledge alone is nevertheless insufficient for professional practice. Knowing *how*

1. Marx W. Wartofsky, *Conceptual Foundations of Scientific Thought* (New York: The Macmillan Co., 1968).

also demands mastery of practice principles, rules, and techniques and requires the exercise of informed judgment in uncertain situations. Skills in making decisions; in solving problems; in individualizing cases and client readiness to use help; in disciplining idiosyncratic style; in operationalizing values; in communicating; and most important, in appreciating the unique effect of cultural, racial, ethnic, class, and other influences, all are part of the knowing *how*. They determine the difference between an amateurish attempt and professional performance. Here again, if we could be sure in our judgment of this aspect of a professional worker's abilities, we would be more comfortable in our selection of a potential helper.

What Must She Be?

We would like to respect a professional not only for what she knows and what she can do but for the kind of person she is. Offhand, this attribute may seem less important than the other two noted, but in critical circumstances it can supersede both in the decision to choose one helper over another.[2] It is hard to assess the importance of a helper's personal value system in relation to the particular service you want rendered. It may be enough that you have a general reassurance that she empathizes with those virtues, duties, and social concerns that you feel are important—in that they can and do influence the relationship you will establish with one another. In addition, you would certainly want some certainty that she is ethical, at least in the performance of her practice. Life provides many examples of skills that are both informed and proficient but are nevertheless misused because

2. Harold Lewis, "Agology, Animation, Conscientization: Implications for Social Work Education in the U.S.A.," *Journal of Education for Social Work* 9, no. 3 (Fall 1973): 31–38.

the interests to be served are not those of the recipient of the service. Nor are ethical behaviors the only characteristics of an individual to be considered. Sensitivity, commitment, caring, and other personal attributes can be absolutely critical in some helping situations and less important in others.

In addition to these personal attributes, it is also helpful that a worker be aware of her own limitations. Knowing the difficulty and duration of her preparation for professional work and understanding how rarely professionals actually achieve the level of skill in knowing and doing that they themselves would ask of any person to whom they might turn for help, she would want to be held accountable for what she does — not only to her peers but also to those of us in trouble who must turn to her for help.

The Agency Worker

With few exceptions, those who seek the services of social workers are neither free to choose who will serve them nor informed enough to select their helpers on the basis of the criteria just discussed. They must almost always turn to social service agencies to obtain social work services. For this reason, agencies must clearly know the attributes they seek in their workers — the consumers of their services must rely on their judgment for assurances otherwise unavailable to them. Of necessity, the wider community's interest in these matters has led to the licensing of agencies and practitioners and the establishment of other monitoring procedures to maintain desirable standards of service. Nevertheless, from the way an agency selects and inducts its staff, from the way it audits and monitors their performance, and from the way it holds them accountable for their activities one can learn still more about the worker who engages in the practice of social work.

Selecting Staff

In recruiting and selecting professional staff, the agency must rely on a limited number of sources for answers to these questions: What does she know? What can she do? What sort of person is she? If an agency hires professionals, it must first seek evidence that certain preparation has occurred. With rare exceptions, the most important measure of such preparation is completion of a program of professional education, which certifies that a candidate has the relevant knowledge, abilities, and personal attributes relevant to her work as a professional helper. Evaluations of previous experience and character references from reputable persons reinforce the evidence of appropriate educational preparation and indicate the candidate's adequacy in motivation and commitment to work that the job entails. Finally, interviews provide immediate and essential evidence of a sort not otherwise available. Where actual performance can be observed, perhaps the most meaningful evidence of all can be obtained. When such evidence is lacking, it is not unusual for an agency to require a probationary period during which performance can be observed and evaluated before a permanent contractual arrangement is made. Thus, an agency applies the criteria for selection in a way rarely available to the consumer of services provided by social workers.

This process, however, throws little light either on the way the worker achieves professional competence or on the role of agencies in helping her gain such competence. To clarify this process we can examine a common occurrence in social service agencies—the induction of a new worker to perform a social work function. In such instances, because the social agency provides the sanction for the worker to engage in practice, it is especially obligated to oversee the quality of her performance. Unlike the acculturated staff member, this worker is somewhat less informed, possibly less skilled, and as yet uninitiated to the agency's value set.

THE INDUCTEE

AN INDUCTEE, if experience is a guide, is likely to be somewhat anxious as she gets started in the new job. She appreciates some direction to help minimize the mistakes she might make because of her own ignorance of agency practice. She wants to carry through her initial contact with recipients of the agency's services in a helpful manner and does not want to deny them benefits from agency services because she herself is not adequately informed.

She quickly discovers that her uncertainties and concerns are not nearly so new to the agency as she is to its practice. Those directly responsible for her induction are equally concerned with the immediate effect of her practice on agency recipients. They quickly inform her about the agency's purpose; about her rights and obligations as its representative; about those of the recipient; about her style in interpersonal relationships and how it relates to the agency's; about this agency's way of providing help when help is needed. She will be reassured in her use of what she does know in the recipient's behalf. Although she may initially welcome this guidance (even as she resents her need to depend on it), she will also find it supportive quickly to socialize to the agency's culture. Being required to get to work on time; to relate to other employees; to listen to instructions and follow them; to organize her job routines and meet her deadlines; to learn what services the agency can offer, what resources are at its disposal, and what policies and procedures govern their availability and use; to relate positively to agency authority (while maintaining a critical stance toward its shortcomings); and not the least important, to represent the agency in the community—all these contribute to her rapid orientation to the work she does.

Knowing and Doing

An inductee could understandably question a requirement that she master what is known about human growth and behavior, about the social environment, or about the history and policies affecting her service as prerequisites for starting with the agency. She could argue that her immediate need would best be served if she only had some systematic introduction to her job responsibilities — including some guidance to help bolster her shaky status as a new helper. Gaps in her knowledge in these larger areas could then be a matter for future consideration. The need for practical suggestions to be put to immediate use should take precedence. In this respect, the inductee will be anticipating the usual course of induction into practice as it is experienced by every beginning student in a professional school of social work.[3]

The inductee usually finds that the agency is prepared to meet her needs. In fact, much of what she is seeking in initial direction may already be codified in an agency manual of policies and procedures. In the absence of a manual, it will be provided through inservice training and through contact with more experienced colleagues. The agency will also

3. For a brief, thoughtful description of this induction process in the agency, see Martha Moscrop, *In-Service Training for Agency Practice* (Toronto: University of Toronto Press, 1958), pp. 160–62; and Carol A. Meyer, *Staff Development in Public Welfare Agencies* (New York: Columbia University Press, 1966), pp. 117–51. For examples of induction in field work for students in schools of social work, see the classic study by Bertha Copen Reynolds, *Learning and Teaching in the Practice of Social Work* (New York: Farrar and Rinehart, 1942); as well as Charlotte Towle, *The Learner in Education for the Professions* (Chicago: University of Chicago Press, 1954); Virginia Robinson, *The Development of a Professional Self: Selected Writings 1930–68* (New York: AMS Press, 1978); and a collection of essays relevant to this process, *Social Work Supervision* ed. Carlton E. Munson (New York: The Free Press, 1979).

designate a senior staff member to oversee her work and consult with her regularly about her performance on the job. A good manual of agency policies and procedures will provide the inductee with her first comprehensive view of what the agency administration expects her to know and do; a concise summary of the agency's rules for action.

Nevertheless, adapting to the agency's way of work will probably prove demanding. The agency's administrator will want her to assimilate ideas and procedures that will shape her personal style to the agency's. An inductee who supposedly knows all about the meaning and theory of time and has mastered the literature on interpersonal relationships will be less than convincing in her claim to knowledge if she is frequently late for appointments or if others find it difficult and irritating to work with her.

More important than ability to understand the job and to master the requirements of codified routines is the inductee's willingness to accept and work within the framework set by the agency's ideology, as it is manifest in its policies and procedures. Such willingness may call for judgments that initially must be based on beliefs that are put forth by the agency but are not necessarily self-evident truths from the inductee's viewpoint. Although the inductee may accept the proposition that her own career will prosper to the degree that she serves a useful social purpose, the function she performs (with infrequent exceptions) occurs under the auspices of a social service agency — and the policies and procedures of that agency will significantly determine the value framework within which both agency and inductee must function. The inductee's usefulness to society must necessarily be inextricably bound up with that of the agency that employs her; and her self-interest, one expects, will prompt her to accept the belief statements of that agency — on the assumption that those responsible for the work of the agency, like herself, want it to succeed in achieving its goals and therefore seek to be guided by truths whose consequences in practice have been evaluated.

Organizations, such as social agencies, have been subjected to systematic study by a variety of disciplines; and a number of useful generalizations about their operations have been proposed.[4] Let us assume that the inductee is somewhat informed about the findings of such studies and that those directing the work of the agency are at least as well informed. She has already concluded that scholarly interest in organizational analysis and bureaucratic structures has some significance for her work. For example, how her own purposes and values (and those of the profession) fare in the context of a bureaucracy is a matter of no little concern to her. In the scholarly literature, she may detect a tendency to focus on the tension-producing conflict between personal, professional, and bureaucratic ideologies; but it does not surprise her—this conflict feels familiar.

Fortunately, the immediate pressures of the job will direct the inductee away from such generalizations about organizations and bureaucracies and toward learning about *this* organization and *its* bureaucracy; *its* goals and *its* objectives. She wants to experience its work routines, to discover how its policies and procedures are developed and how its program is directed and supported. She finds that the agency's willingness to accept her limited background is a welcome consider-

4. See, for example, Amitai Etzioni, ed., *A Sociological Reader on Complex Organizations,* 2d ed. (New York: Holt, Rinehart & Winston, 1969); Simon Slavin, ed., *Social Administration: The Management of the Social Services* (New York: Haworth Press and the Council on Social Work Education, 1978); Felice Davidson Perlmutter and Simon Slavin, eds., *Leadership in Social Administration* (Philadelphia: Temple University Press, 1980); Rosemary C. Sarri and Yeheskel Hasenfeld, eds., *The Management of Human Services* (New York: Columbia University Press, 1978); and Herman D. Stein, ed., *Organization and the Human Services: Cross-Disciplinary Reflections* (Philadelphia: Temple University Press, 1981).

ation, in exchange for which she is expected to accept concise and explicit directives for behaving according to agency expectations and in a style congenial to its pattern of work.

Personal Beliefs

Turning to the manual, or its equivalent, the inductee may find her orientation to the agency facilitated. She may have read elsewhere that an organization's ideology serves to preserve its internal unity and that challenges to this ideology are recognized by the bureaucracy as a threat to its unity.[5] She may not yet realize that her personal resistance to certain routines specified in the manual is a concrete instance of such a challenge.

It is not unusual for a manual to require that she give up a cherished style of her own, thus restricting her self-determination and posing a threat to her personal integrity. She is expected to conform, to be responsive to the needs of the bureaucracy, and to trust that such conformity on her part will make her more efficient and effective. At this level of procedural norms expressed in required behavior, the inductee will quickly come to know the meaning of the agency's ideology and her agreements and differences with it. Direct experience will provide empirical evidence to support such knowledge, and its similarity to the experiences reported by her peers and mentors will reinforce her own.

For the inductee, this evidence will appear to support beliefs; and it will more than likely be claimed as personal knowledge that others undergoing similar experiences can appreciate. In this context, reports of what has personally been experienced are nonjudgmental — they are not intended to predict. If the inductee takes her personal experience as

5. Barrows Dunham, *Heroes and Heretics* (New York: Dell Publishing Co., Delta Books, 1968), pp. 12–24.

evidence about objective phenomena and compares the statements of her peers with reports in the literature about similarly experienced personal knowledge to find evidence of the same phenomena, she will be venturing a judgment whose probable truth is then subject to test by procedures that meet acceptable standards for establishing credibility. Predictions based on such judgments must be empirically verifiable by their consequences. Both belief statements expressed as personal reports and statements that imply predictive accuracy may concern the same phenomena, both may be true statements, but only the latter offers a judgment about objective phenomena that requires evidence, other than the reported belief, to achieve credibility.

Obviously, personal belief statements are not without significance in shaping the performance of an inductee. By definition, they constitute her personal orientation and provide the color and contour of her style. The very fact that an inductee both acknowledges such beliefs and assumes that others undergoing similar experiences will report similar beliefs, prepares her to appreciate the implications of recipients' beliefs that may otherwise escape her attention. If meeting agency requirements (i.e., accepting agency beliefs) produces tension for the worker, does it not do the same for the recipients of agency services? If the worker's personal style is threatened by agency style, what does this imply for the recipient, whose freedom of choice may be more restricted? In short, the inductee's personal experience should alert her to the tensions and fears of recipients who seek the help of an agency.

Beliefs derived from personal experience are statements of fact to the extent that they describe subjective evaluations.[6] Predictive statements, in contrast, proffer explanations

6. Michael Polanyi, *Personal Knowledge* (Chicago: University of Chicago Press, 1958), pp. 17, 255–57.

directly supportable by observations of their consequences. For the inductee, such support is inseparable from the practice experiences that produce it. She is hardly likely to accept other persons' interpretations and action-directives about her own beliefs. Nor will she readily accept explanations of her predictive statements that contradict her own observations. For her, alternate explanations must be established as truth through acceptable criteria of proof.

As the inductee seeks to meet the requirements of her immediate supervisor, what she is expected to know turns the inquiry directly on herself as helper. It becomes increasingly difficult to separate beliefs from predictive statements. She will often be asked to consider her personal evaluation of her own reaction to some phenomena—in which case she is in fact being asked to state her beliefs about her beliefs. Her responses (excluding deliberate distortions or failures in communication) are offered as nonjudgmental self-reports. Should her supervisor judge her responses to be faulty—that is, inappropriate to the predictive explanations objective phenomena are expected to promote—the supervisor may try to convince the worker that her responses should change. For the inductee, her beliefs ought not be questioned as 'true' or 'false' since they are personal reports. They may be questioned as 'right' or 'wrong' as assertions about values, not as assertions about knowledge. Should the inductee challenge the supervisor's views of right and wrong, their dialogue can move from a discussion of opinion to consideration of fact only if the inductee's beliefs are reformulated as predictive statements. Seeking how-to-do-it guidelines, the inductee is thus led to consider how-to-do-it procedures as well.

How does the inductee come to know her own beliefs and appreciate their influence on the practice decisions she makes? In addition to self-evaluations, she may be helped to a deeper realization of her beliefs and their implications through the efforts of an agency mentor. Practice demands that an inductee make unavoidable choices and suffer their consequences. Despite all the choices previously experienced in agency practice, the inductee must always face choices not anticipated in existing policies and procedures. Such choices involving unknowns must rely on the inductee's beliefs. Having to make such choices forces the inductee to realize that beliefs, her own in particular, directly affect actions.

In an effort to open her to questions that might reveal her to herself, the inductee's supervisor may direct her to review the literature. Reading in psychology and sociology is ordinarily suggested, but excursions into great literature — novels, biographies, plays, essays, and poetry — can similarly provide the inductee with self-perception of an unusually acute quality. Such readings may deepen her appreciation of the ways personal beliefs influence action and style. Of equal importance, the inductee may learn that she brings more strength to her assignment than she thought she possessed in this area of personal knowledge.

The inductee will thus be called upon to acquire a considerable body of knowledge and values. Because she will also be called upon to exercise judgments in uncertain situations, she needs considerable self-awareness as well. The nature of the work to be done (and the conditions under which it will be done) realistically suggest the need for a formal mechanism whereby appropriate induction into practice may take place.

What has been said of the inductee, then, holds equally true for the experienced professional, but at a more sophisticated level. The areas of uncertainty; the gaps in knowledge; the doubts about effectiveness; the difficulties with organizational restraints; the tension between personal, professional, and agency beliefs; and insistent need to "know thyself," all remain a part of the burden a worker in this profession carries as a requirement for the job. What changes with professional preparation and experience is the way these requirements are met—the professional worker being competent to exercise more options than are available to the inductee.

The reason for providing so detailed a picture of the worker in the social agency should be fairly obvious: Social work is a socialized profession.[7] Its practitioners, with few exceptions, work for social agencies. Their clients usually come seeking the services of the agencies that employ them and in that way come into contact with them. If one is to understand the social worker, one must see her as a functionary of an organization or miss a good deal of the range and nature of her role and function. Much of what she must know and do is influenced by where and for whom she works, by the tasks she is expected to perform, and by the recipients of her service. The induction of the worker into the agency serves both to acculurate her to the social work profession and to help her to learn how to do her job.

THE RECIPIENT

NO DISCUSSION of the worker is complete without some consideration of the recipient, whose need makes service possible. Each of the elements of work—the condition to be altered, the goal to be achieved, the resource to be expended—influences the work of the recipient. Much of the dynamic that invests service with its power to transform results from the views that both worker and recipient bring to their engagement. All approaches to practice provide in their formulation for the active participation of the recipient in shaping the service process.[8] The importance of the

7. A.M. Car-Saunders and P.A. Wilson, *The Professions* (Oxford: At the Clarendon Press, 1933), pp. 451–57.

8. William J. Reid and Laura Epstein, *Task Centered Practice* (New York: Columbia University Press, 1978), pp. 138–78; Helen Harris Perlman, *Social Casework: A Problem Solving Process* (Chicago: University of Chicago Press, 1957), pp. 58–63; Florence Hollis, *Casework: A*

recipient's contribution to the creation of a service in which he participates is considered in detail in later chapters.

Condition to Be Changed

It is not uncommon for the recipient and the worker to agree on the circumstances that make service necessary. They may also agree on steps that might be taken to change these circumstances. Nevertheless, the worker's understanding of the

---

Psychosocial Therapy, 2d ed. (New York: Random House, 1974), pp. 28–35; William Schwartz and Zolba Serspio, eds., *The Practice of Group Work* (New York: Columbia University Press, 1971), pp. 3–24; Ruth E. Smalley, *Theory of Social Work Practice* (New York: Columbia University Press, 1967), pp. 167–75; Ruth R. Middleman and Gale Goldberg, *Social Service Delivery: A Structural Approach to Social Work Practice* (New York: Columbia University Press, 1974), pp. 32–53; Howard Goldstein, *Social Work Practice: A Unitary Approach* (Columbia: University of South Carolina Press, 1973), pp. 120–52; Allen Pincus and Anne Minahan, *Social Work Practice: Model and Method* (Itasca, Illinois: F.E. Peacock, 1973), pp. 56–63; Max Siporin, *Introduction to Social Work Practice* (New York: Macmillan Co., 1975), pp. 78–185; Judith Nelson, *Communication Theory and Social Work Practice* (Chicago: University of Chicago Press, 1980), pp. 89–112; Alex Gitterman and Carol B. Gerwain, *The Life Model of Social Work Practice* (New York: Columbia University Press, 1980), pp. 15–17; Carol H. Meyer, *Social Work Practice: The Changing Landscape,* 2d ed. (New York: Free Press, 1976), pp. 169–203; Joel Fischer, *Effective Casework Practice: An Eclectic Approach* (New York: McGraw Hill Book Co., 1978), pp. 13–15; Joel Fischer and Harvey L. Grochros, *Planned Behavior Change: Behavior Modification in Social Work* (New York: Free Press, 1975), pp. 109–12; Sheldon D. Rose, *Group Therapy: A Behavioral Approach* (Englewood Cliffs, N.J.: Prentice Hall, 1972), pp. 4–6; Robert W. Roberts and Robert Nee, eds., *Theories of Social Casework* (Chicago: University of Chicago Press, 1970); Robert W. Roberts and Helen Norther, eds., *Theories of Social Work with Groups* (New York, Columbia University Press, 1976); Francis J. Turner, ed., *Social Work Treatment: Interlocking Theoretical Approaches,* 2d ed. (New York: Free Press, 1979); Edward John Thomas, ed., *Behavioral Modification Procedures* (Chicago: Aldine Publishing Co., 1974).

condition to be altered often differs from the recipient's. For example, a recipient may not perceive emotional and physical deprivation and inappropriate behavior where a worker sees lack of affection, inadequacy of housing and dress, and neglect of a child. Such differences clearly involve more than simple conflicts of perception.

In part, these differences result from different life experiences, different standards of evaluation, and different cultural frames of reference. They also reflect a disparity between what the recipient expects from the worker and her agency and what the worker expects from the recipient as a participant in the service.

Goal

For example, each may propose a different answer to this question: Whose goal shall be worked toward in the service transaction, the recipient's or the worker's? It can be argued that the proper goal will evolve through the interchange between worker and recipient. When this is so, the unmet need is defined by the service exchange and is mutually acceptable. When this occurs, both parties avoid imposed intentions, and both worker and recipient become free to develop a useful service. Unhappily, because the recipient often seeks help precisely because of an inability to clarify goals and objectives, he or she brings to the helping relationship all the doubts and feelings of diminished hope. In these circumstances, the agency's goals and objectives, as interpreted by the worker, are likely to overwhelm those of the recipient. The exchange between them will in all likelihood be more of a one-way street—conditioning the recipient to the worker's intentions rather than the other way around. Even if the exchange is ideally conceived of as a meeting of equals, the unequal power of the parties to the relationship will dictate the outcome. In any typical service encounter in direct practice, the power is on the side of the worker. In community work or in situations where the recipient controls the allocations of resources, it may more often favor the recipient.[9] Such differences in the power relationship necessarily influence the choice of goals and objectives in the provision of service.

Resources

The recipient is interested in knowing how the personal resources brought to the service transaction will be expended and what this expenditure will bring in return. Initially, the recipient is unlikely to see the worker's assessment of need and choice of interventive procedure as a source of help. For the recipient, the requirements resulting from the worker's activities often appear to represent the price of admission to the service. The cost entailed is worth the expenditure if it promises more than other investments of the same energies. This observation assumes, of course, that the recipient is free to choose and is not acting under the compulsion of some authority in engaging in the service. In the latter instance, the choice may be based more on a desire to avoid punishment than on a motivation to achieve maximum use of available personal resources.[10]

The service exchange can be socially and psychologically beneficial for both worker and recipient. The recipient will then sustain the relationship so long as it appears to yield a positive cost/benefit ratio. When the reverse is true, the reci-

9. Patricia Yancey Martin, "A Critical Analysis of Power in Professional-Client Relations," *Aretê* 6, no. 3 (Spring 1981): 35–48; Nina Toren, *Social Work: The Case of a Semi-Profession* (Beverly Hills, Calif.: Sage Publications, 1972), pp. 95–128, 189–223; Frances Fox Piven and Richard A. Cloward, *Regulating the Poor: The Function of Public Welfare* (New York: Pantheon Books, 1971), pp. 38–41.

10. Shankar A. Yelaja, ed., *Authority and Social Work* (Toronto: University of Toronto Press, 1971), pp. 171–298.

pient will terminate if free to do so. When a recipient is compelled to participate in a relationship he thinks is negative, however, many difficult ethical dilemmas confront the worker. If worker and recipient work together in a resource exchange, altering the condition in the intended direction becomes more and more likely.

THE PRODUCT

SOCIAL WORK SERVICES have distinctive attributes as commodities.[11] In the past, they were rarely available on a competitive basis. Usually, each service is to be had from only one source in a community. Even when associated with tangible social services, such as daycare, homemaker care, or foster care, social work services are labor intensive. The average recipient finds it difficult to evaluate their quality and to appreciate what constitutes an appropriate quantity to meet a specific need. Most social work services are provided by tax-supported sources; rarely are their costs covered by recipient payments.

Social work services materialize in the very act of being rendered. There is no service as such in the resources allocated for their provision, any more than service is latent in the recipient's needs. Only when provider resources and recipient needs join in an actual transaction, does a service, as a commodity, evolve. Thus, unlike most commodities in our economy, social work services exist only in the process of formation — they have no existence apart from it.

11. Harold Lewis, "The Social Service Commodity in the Inflationary 80's" (Paper presented at Family Service Association of America Workshop for Directors of Professional Services, Toronto, Ontario, 1980); David M. Austin, "The Political Economy of Social Benefit Organizations: Redistributive Services of Merit Goods," in *Organization and the Human Services* ed. Herman Stein (Philadelphia: Temple University Press, 1981), pp. 37–89.

For this reason, one cannot inventory social work services in the traditional sense: One cannot go to a bin and count how many of these and how many of those are on hand to meet current demand. Although available resources suggests that a potential is available for providing various services, it hardly constitutes a count of the services themselves; and the availability of a resource offers no assurance that it will be used in a transaction that produces a service. Unhappily, the transient nature of service allows it to disappear without too much notice of its absence on the part of persons other than those directly involved in its production and consumption. Inventories of unsold cars convey a far more dramatic message of economically unproductive policies and practices than does the disappearance of transactions that produce social work services.

This commodity is short lived: the transaction both creates it and absorbs it in toto. After the fact, the only evidence that the commodity was created and consumed is a depletion of resources and a change in recipient condition. Thus, if the quality of the commodity is to be directly evaluated, what transpires during the exchange of provisions for needs must be observed in process. Evaluations after the fact inevitably encounter the complex problem of isolating particular effects in situations involving matrixes of causal influences. Guaranteeing the quality of such a service is difficult: Unlike the faulty brake or slipping transmission, a service cannot be recalled by the manufacturer for correction of a fault. Inasmuch as there is no clear product that can be demonstrated to be defective, it is more convenient to fault the program that provides the service than the particular social work methods that are used to create it.[12]

12. Harold Lewis, "Developing Programs Responsive to New Knowledge and Values," in *Evaluation of Social Intervention* ed. Edward J. Mullen, James R. Dumpson, and Associates (San Francisco: Josey-Bass, 1972), pp. 72–73.

Like all commodities, social work services have *use value* as well as *exchange value*. As with any human service, the use value is largely determined by recipient's judgments of costs relative to the satisfactions obtained by participating in its creation. The exchange value, on the other hand, relies more heavily on the judgments of providers. Determining what alternate uses can be made of an equal investment of resources largely fixes its exchange value. From the recipient's perspective, the better the quality for equal cost, the higher the use value one can assign to the commodity. From the provider's perspective, the less costly the resource (other things being equal) the greater the exchange value. Given these considerations, it is important to note that the persons creating the social work service—the worker and the recipient—are most often dependent on relatively disinterested parties for the crucial decisions about the quality and quantity of service to be subsidized.

Finally, it is important to recognize the logic that applies to analyzing and understanding this commodity's relationship to the satisfaction of specified needs. In all but a few instances, the intention of social work services is to enhance the potential for constructive choices on the part of their recipients. A major objective for the worker and outcome for the recipient is meeting a need in such a way that the recipient's dependency on the service will be diminished as far as possible if he is confronted with a similar need in the future. The service is thus expected not only to have a fixed, determined effect as an outcome but also to improve the recipient's capacity for coping in a wide range of social functioning areas. None of our evaluative procedures, based as they are on statistical aggregates of individual units, can tell us what will happen in a particular case served, or in the next case to be served.

Beyond this probability issue, which the literature has discussed in detail, lurks another and more fundamental probability issue. When they seek help, recipients bring to the transaction a variety of potentials in behavior, reasoning, valuing, and the like—all interdependent. As a result of the service, the distribution of these potentials should change in a way that can provide some measure of the nature and scope of the impact of the service. The most demanding aspects of a service transaction, those for which professional social work skills are most clearly required, fall in this problematic area: the objective measurement of change and potential change. In fact, these potentials have yet to be adequately described. For example, when does self-awareness, which may be an important indicator of a person's potential for constructive interpersonal relationships, become self-preoccupation, an indicator of the opposite potential?[13] To arrive at operational definitions of self-awareness and self-preoccupation we need to know much more about these qualities than we now do. Moreover, given the bio-psycho-social influences on their development, measuring such quixotic qualities can prove as futile as counting melting ice cubes—the inevitable result is watered-down statistics.

Complicating the task of measurement is the intentional nature of social work service. Service is normally shaped by its creators to achieve particular effects. It would be necessary first to determine what was to be altered in relation to nontargeted potentials and second to understand their interactions before one could conclude whether a particular intervention produced a particular change in potential for acceptable social functioning.

These unique attributes of the product of social work practice—taken together with the roles of both the worker and the recipient in producing a social work service—

12. Florence Wexler Vigilante, "Self-Preoccupation As a Predictor of Performance in Graduate Social Work Education" (D.S.W. Diss., Yeshiva University, 1980) attempts to operationalize these concepts.

constitute a complex conceptual problem for any worker seeking to achieve skill in her performance. It is not surprising that workers come to rely on powerful intellectual tools to assist them in their practice. In Part 2, I describe the tools most frequently employed and relate each to the level of skill reflected in its appropriate use.

»» ««

PART II

The Elements of Skill

CHAPTER THREE

»» ««

Intellectual Tools

THE PRINCIPAL intellectual task in professional practice is the blending of means and ends, of technique and purpose. The basic intellectual tools available to facilitate this task are rules and principles, which make it easier to incorporate the lessons of action in guidelines for practice. Rules and principles also respond to changing preferences with respect to knowledge and values as they are simultaneously informed by theory and justified by ethical imperatives. Accordingly, in this chapter, I have made it a rule, wherever it serves to clarify, to cite an example from practice. This rule is justified by the principle that where my intention is to demonstrate their utility, the more general and abstract formulations must be ·buttressed by specific instances that illustrate their application.

It is important to appreciate the dynamic nature of rules and principles. The practice of social work is never static. It is constantly responding to economic and political pressures and to changes in the knowledge base on which it operates. The driving force penetrating the relationship of means and ends nevertheless assures the profession that its practice will remain relevant to a society that is itself in flux.[1]

Rules likewise remain in flux, so long as the directives they

1. Harold Lewis, "The Cause in Function," *Journal of the Otto Rank Association* 2, no. 2 (Winter 1976–77): 18–25.

enunciate and the commands they convey continue to undergo change. The unity of directive and command—of means and ends—expressed in rules is temporary. In the course of time, tensions arise as the directives and commands contained in rules are altered, first to reflect changes in what is known (thus affecting means) and second to accommodate changes in the social and political context in which they are applied (thus influencing ends). As the tensions contained in rules are resolved, the rules themselves change to assure their relevance for the practice they help shape.

From a set of rules, one can identify the principles that inform and justify them. Changing rules compel changes in principles or reflect changes required by principles.

Principles also remain in flux. Because the propositions contained in principles represent the current state of practice knowledge, they necessarily are altered as more becomes known. The ethical commendations contained in principles *(should, ought, must)* change more slowly. Nevertheless, as values shift and as ethical imperatives intended to realize these values in action begin to reflect these shifts, the commendations embedded in principles also change. As is the case with rules, the unity of the propositions and commendations contained in principles is temporary. As theory and ethics change, as what we know and believe changes, principles continue to evolve to assure their continued relevance to practice. See Figure 2.

RULES AND PRINCIPLES

IT IS ESSENTIAL to understand how rules facilitate actions; how in a professional practice they help the worker exercise control over events and situations. Unlike the laws of theoretical sciences, which describe and explain, rules give direction and purpose to action. Rules are not attributes of

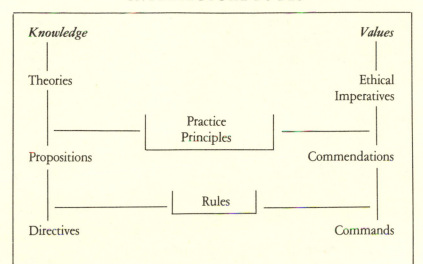

Figure 2. Hierarchical ordering of concepts: knowlege and values. A *rule* combines a directive and a command, providing instruction for appropriate action. Rules *structure* a practice. A *principle* combines a propositional statement and a commendation providing guidelines for appropriate action. Principles structure programs and *justify* a practice.

the processes they generate, they are mind made. Thus, even when we distill from a set of actions the probable rules that helped to shape it, what we identify tells us more about what went on in the mind of the worker than it does about the products of her work.

It is not surprising, then, to find rules serving as basic tools in the mental work of a profession. Nor is it unexpected to discover how such relatively simple directives help generate a very complex form — the practice principle.

Rules

Rules guide the social worker in her practice. For example, she is told to respect the privacy of her clients and to recognize the uniqueness of each individual and each case. These simple instructions, if followed, will significantly influence the work involved in providing a social work service. In combination, rules suggest a complex practice principle — in the first instance, the principle of confidentiality. Of course, as every practitioner knows, simply following rules can be anything but simple.

The pervasive influence of the agency milieu on the character of social work is evident from the manner in which rules shape the actions of social workers as agency employees.

Those responsible for supervising the work of an agency are anxious to assure acceptable standards of professional practice and organizational effectiveness. Toward these ends, they carefully husband the ongoing experience of the staff. As a result, an agglomeration of *do's* and *don'ts* accrues to the agency's store of tested procedures. These are then usually codified, assembled in manuals, taught in orientation programs, and communicated by program supervisors.

The following statements, which are taken from a manual developed by a child welfare agency for its protective service staff, illustrate various categories of rules and how the rules in each catagory provide the worker with directives for action in a specific situation.[2] For each rule, a further breakdown is provided to identify the tasks to be performed in the implementation of the rule so as to highlight the action-oriented directives contained in each rule.

Five elements that enter into the performance of a task are likely to be codified into rules. They usually give rise to direc-

---

2. Ben Ami Gelin and Julius A. Jahn, "Research Design," in "Designing More Effective Protective Services: Appendix," ed. Harold Lewis, Julius Jahn, Shankar Yalaija, and Ben Ami Gelin (Philadelphia: University of Pennsylvania School of Social Work Research Center, 1967), pp. 4–5; see also Sr. Mary Paul Janchill, *Guidelines to Decision-Making in Child Welfare* (New York: The Human Services Workshop, 1981), pp. 5–7, for examples of guiding practice principles that provide a justifying framework for rules.

tives intended to accomplish the following objectives: *(1)* order activities in time; *(2)* assure coverage of substantive content; *(3)* assure inclusion of appropriate persons and organizations in process; *(4)* encourage uniform adherence to agency policies where critical practice decisions must be made; and *(5)* provide evidence of work done, assuring accountability. The rules presented here have been chosen to illustrate each of these elements.

RULE 1 A conference with the referring agency is required before contacting the family if there is a question of appropriateness of the referral or necessity to clarify a complex of services to the family that would enable the agency to make a more appropriate decision about action or give better service.

Tasks

Determine if there is a question of appropriateness of the referral. If yes, plan a conference with the referring agency to clarify the question. Plan contact with the family to take place after the conference with the referring agency.

RULE 2 In opening a case, the intake worker makes clear to parent(s) the specific areas of neglect identified, informs the parent(s) of the agency's responsibility in protecting the children, and determines whether the parent(s) are sufficiently concerned to use the agency's services.

Tasks

Note the specific areas of neglect and specify evidence of such neglect.

Explain to the parent(s) the agency's desire to help the family achieve adequate care.

Note any evidence of efforts by parent(s) toward

beginning improvement in areas of child care where neglect was evidenced.

Seek evidence of parent(s) willingness to accept agency's condition for help.

RULE 3 Both parents should be seen when children are living with them both or when both are active in the children's lives.

Tasks

Determine if the children are living with both parents or if both are active in the children's lives.

Plan contacts with the family to assure seeing both parents in the course of continuing service.

RULE 4 A case is always refered to court by petition when

1. neglect or abuse exists and the parent(s) or guardian is unable or unwilling to improve care to a safer level;
2. agency service is refused and the nature of the report of neglect and/or abuse indicates that children are in danger;
3. parents want placement for a child but are unable to sustain a voluntary placement process, and agency agrees there is need for placement;
4. court order is needed in order to bring a child into care or to hold the child there once admitted;
5. a child in the case will need continued placement or return home on protection;
6. a child without legal guardian is admitted to care.

Tasks

Determine if one or more of the above conditions are present in the case.

List the conditions present for inclusion in the record.

Determine if a petition is to be filed.

RULE 5 Follow the opening summary as described in the manual in all cases and record the information obtained in the case record. (Included in the summary are the following:

1. Date recorded;
2. Neglect reported-date;
3. Family composition;
4. Income;
5. Contacts with the family;
6. Information from other sources;
7. Neglect and evaluation;
8. Plans with other agencies;
9. Information re planning with family.)

Tasks

Obtain necessary information to complete opening summary. Record opening summary information into case record.

Typically, these rules define a practice. They are intended to instruct the worker in how to engage in it.[3] The worker understands their purpose, and her understanding is constantly reenforced by reminders from supervisors and from the systematized procedures established by the agency to report changes in these rules.[4] A worker starting in the agency will quickly learn to accept these rules in the performance of her function since she may be held responsible for failing to follow them. Although she may argue that various possible activities are equally encompassable by the same rule, so long as she accepts the agency's practice, following the rules remains the test of adherence to the agency's re-

3. John Rawls, "Two Concepts of Rules," *The Philosophical Review* 64, no. 1 (January 1955): 3–33.
4. Carlton E. Munson, ed., *Social Work Supervision* (New York: The Free Press, 1979).

quirements. Should she challenge the rules, she would in effect be questioning the agency's practice.

As the illustrations make clear, such rules offer no guidance for making decisions in uncertain situations, where a worker must appeal to less specific but more encompassing guiding principles. Each case must be made to fit the rule, or the rule must be qualified in such a way as to provide for the unanticipated elements introduced by the case. Exceptions to the rule are to be avoided.

Clearly, these rules are addressed to workers in their capacity as agents of an agency who are called upon to perform its work. The restraint such rules place upon the worker constitutes a price exacted in exchange for the support they provide her in her practice.

There is therefore a need for rules that justify some discretion on the part of the worker.[5] This is especially important in a practice where unanticipated occurrences must be acted upon in the absence of relevant rules. Such enabling rules are most often manifest in the provision of channels and means that assure the regular review of an agency's purpose, function, policies, structure, procedures, and services. Through such channels, the worker can call the agency's attention to changes in the community's attitudes, resources, and needs and to changes in its own program and clientele that not only necessitate the enactment of new rules or the modification or elimination of existing rules but also call for alternatives in objectives, standards, methods, and services. It often happens that such channels are either unavailable or unable to function appropriately. In such cases, the worker who finds the prevalent rules inappropriate must appeal to the higher

5. Rino J. Patti, "Organizational Resistance and Change: The View from Below," in *Social Administration*. ed. Simon Slavin (New York: Haworth Press, 1978), pp. 541–56.

level of professional authority incorporated in principles of professional practice that the rules appear to violate.[6]

Characteristics of Rules

Rules make no explicit claim to knowledge or belief. Moreover, rules make no reference to goals. As directives for action, they spell out the process the worker is expected to initiate, sustain, and terminate in her practice. Although it is sometimes assumed that rules, taken as a set of action guides, are consistent with the values and knowledge that in turn justify an agency's program, whether this is in fact the case must be determined empirically. It can be observed, however, that dissatisfaction with the services of an agency frequently centers upon evidence that rules neither implement its purported purposes nor follow the theory used to explain the agency's practice.[7]

A rule is most helpful when it is least ambiguous, least demanding of judgment in its application, and most clearly and quickly associated with the situations to which it applies. These observations suggest what is apparent in practice: Rules are likely to be followed in situations where there is little uncertainty for the worker. Because it stores only limited information and fires an almost instantaneous command to an appropriate inquiry, a rule is most subject to habituation. The efficiency of any rule as an action guide derives from its specificity to a particular situation and its frequent application makes it routine and increasingly easy to use. But overuse can also desensitize the worker to possible misapplication of the rule in practice.

6. George Brager and Stephen Holloway, *Changing Human Service Organizations* (New York: The Free Press, 1978), pp. 1–28.

7. Lewis et al., "Designing Protective Services," pp. 53–61.

Learning Rules

Initially, a worker needs rules to learn quickly and easily what is required of her on the job. In a helping profession, rules appear to be taught most effectively by case example, and through other forms of modeling behavior.[8] But professional rules are not reducible to automatic response directives, since they require some mental storage of information in order to facilitate their recovery for use.

Whenever mental storage must precede recovery and such storage and recovery require nonprogrammed judgment, professional questioning must occur. For a learner who lacks practical experiences, composing appropriate questions is almost impossible without some model associated with particular rules. For the worker, such relevant models suggest how a question may be composed, teach her to recognize a class of similar compositions, and identify common elements characterizing the class. These common elements in turn index the applicable rule for recovery. For this reason, it is not necessary, in practice, to compose questions on the basis of everything that sense data provide. Discrimination of the key elements permits the worker to compose the question that can enter the memory and recover the relevant rule.

The fewer the elements needed to recover a rule, the shorter the interval between observation and action. This habituating quality of rule-governed behavior (and the danger of desensitizing it poses) warns us against the

---

8. Social work education has always relied on field learning for the induction of students into social work practice by enabling them to render service to clients in the context of actual agency work. The field instructor uses the actual case both to teach the rules and to teach the student how to use herself in implementing those rules. For an overview, see Louis Lowy, Leonard M. Bloksberg, and Jerbert J. Walberg, *Integrative Learning and Teaching in Schools of Social Work* (New York: Association Press, 1971), pp. 61–94.

mechanical application of rules. Learning rules without reference to principles can result in unprincipled practice — even though rules are conscientiously, if not consciously, applied.

Changing the Rules

Reasons for changing the rules vary, but they always involve issues of means and ends. When the directive contained in a rule promotes an ineffective intervention, doubts about what is known must follow. Such doubts both inhibit action and precipitate questions concerning the usefulness of the practice. Where the command contained in a rule prompts adherence to the rule even in situations where such adherence appears to defeat program goals (even if it appears to achieve short-term agency objectives), action is similarly inhibited. In either case, practice generates tensions by exposing the uneven development of the means and ends implicit in the rule. Such tensions prompt workers to challenge the rule and appeal to principle. When a sufficient number of rules justified by the same guiding principle are questioned, the principle itself is cast into doubt. The following cases suggest the significance of such inner-developed stimuli in changing the rules.

In an agency serving families charged with child neglect, the worker is directed to "inform the client *in the initial contact* why you have contacted the family: what the agency's responsibility is in cases of this sort, and what services the agency is prepared to provide." This rule is justified as a directive on the grounds that systematic study has shown that it prompts clients into making more effective use of the service. The command in this rule is justified on the grounds that a family has the right to know why an agency is intruding into its life and violating its privacy and independence. A study of efforts to apply this rule, however, found that the client was often unable to take in such information during the first two contacts with the worker.[9] The psychological impact of the charge leveled against the family was so traumatic that it blocked out what the worker was saying about the nature of the service offered. To be useful, the rule had to be modified so as to allow for as many as three contacts to communicate what was originally expected to be shared in one. In this case, the directive (means) side of the rule had to change while the command (ends) side did not.

The reverse is a common experience in agencies seeking to serve the most disadvantaged persons needing access to their resources. The rule may state: "Eligible clients shall be served in the order in which their requests are received, until resources are exhausted." The directive (means) side is based on evidence that such a procedure will minimize value judgments about who shall be preferred in granting access to a service when not all can be served. The command (ends) side is based on the principle of distributive justice that prohibits discrimination in allocating resources on any basis other than identified need. Practice, however, provides evidence that the most disadvantaged are also usually the least likely to know about the availability of the service, the procedure for gaining access to it, and the supportive resources that help connect the potential client with the agency. Thus, although the rule appears to work in accordance with the assumptions that direct its application, in practice, adherence to this rule defeats a goal of the agency—to serve the most disadvantaged, who are likely to be the last to apply, often when resources are seriously or totally depleted. In this case, the means work according to expectations but the ends intended are not realized. In catastrophe relief, the rule calls for returning persons affected by catastrophe to a condition as similar as possible to the one they enjoyed prior to the catastrophe.[10]

9. Lewis et al., "Designing Protective Services," pp. 58–61.

10. John A. Nordheimer, "U.S. Disaster Relief and Built-in Bias," *New York Times* (Reprinted in *San Francisco Chronicle*, 13 January 1970).

In this case, both means and ends fail to deliver the service guided by the rule. The directive is clearly appropriate for distributing resources, and the command implies a commitment to a standard of fairness; but in practice, this approach can divert maximum resources to those persons who enjoyed the most adequate condition prior to the catastrophe, and the net effect of the rule is to use community resources to perpetuate inequities. In this case, a change in principle may be needed.

From Rules to Principles

Often, there are no rules readily available to fit a particular situation. It may also appear that an existing rule is inappropriate for the task at hand. In such circumstances, the worker may seek to formulate a new rule, challenge an existing rule, or do both. A challenge is not likely to affect the policies and procedures of an agency if the worker seeks to justify proposed changes on the basis of her practice alone. Something more than evidence that may be idiosyncratic to the worker is needed to generate concern and involvement among agency staff. The worker must demonstrate that agency practice rather than her own needs to change. Inevitably, as evidence from sources other than her own work is accumulated, she will find she must appeal to some overriding principle governing the rules she wishes to alter to find justification of the changes she proposes.

In appealing to a principle to justify a change in rules, the worker is endorsing the agency's program while questioning its practice. She can use both her experience and that of others to argue for the change in rules, while still maintaining the position that such changes are consistent with the intentions of the program. When the practice experience of the worker and her colleagues leads them to challenge an overriding principle, more than the practice is at stake: Both the program and the agency's very existence are being questioned. So long as the worker means only to change the rules, she may be tolerated as a dissenter; but when her focus shifts and she puts a principle into question, her threat will be viewed as heresy. Whereas survival in the agency in the first instance calls for collective staff support for the recommended change, survival in a situation that implies heresy often also requires a constituency outside the agency who can defend the proposed change and influence the agency's governing body and its programs.[11] In a professional practice, principles are obviously more powerful intellectual tools than are rules.

PRINCIPLES

THE FOLLOWING STATEMENTS are illustrative of principles intended as guides to effective rendering of an agency's services:

- The worker *will* strive to assure the recipient the opportunity to choose her own goal and help her to find it.

- The worker *will* focus on the recipient's current problems and immediate involvements with the agency. This *will* include, on the worker's part, recognition of the need to help the recipient to describe and explore her present feelings about her life experience.

Unlike the rules cited previously, these guidelines avoid specification of tasks, providing instead elements to be considered in performing a role. Considerable leeway is assured the worker, who must find her own procedures for enacting the role. As far as the principle is concerned, the how, when, who, and what of practice are to be individualized to meet

11. John Wax, "Developing Social Work Power in a Medical Organization," *Social Work* 13, no. 4 (1968): 62–71.

the circumstances of each service request. The principle asks only that due regard be given the requirements of its directives. Unlike rules, these principles are clearly *not* intended to provide uniformity and control over practice, being formulated rather so as to allow maximum freedom of choice and innovation in their application.

These two principles provide evidence of how propositions and preferences are combined to provide guidelines for practice. Each assumes that in order to achieve the objectives and goals of practice, such and such must be done.[12] If the intention (will) is removed from each statement, there remains a propositional formulation that may be true or false. For example, the first statement implies that the recipient can make maximum use of agency resource when she is given the opportunity to choose her own goal and helped to find it when necessary. This proposition can be or hopefully will in time be specified operationally and subjected to empirical investigation. It offers the possibility of determining if as a predictive assertion it warrants acceptance as a 'truth.' Such propositions are the essential building blocks of the knowledge claimed by the profession, and it is not difficult to see why this is so. Any design intended to test such a proposition, while often difficult to achieve, can include both the contingent variables associated with the context of agency practice and the intervening variables evidenced in the worker's activities to elicit findings useful in guiding social work practice. Of course, the dependent variables (outcome measures) and the independent variables (agency resources offered by the worker, agency expectations of the recipient, recipient's request) can also be studied without including the effects of such contingent and intervening variables; but the

12. Herbert A. Simon, *Administrative Behavior: A Study of Administrative Processes in Administrative Organizations* (New York: Free Press, 1957), pp. 248–53.

knowlege derived from a study that omits these variables will not be immediately usable in social work practice.

For example, the degree to which enough time to explore the recipient's goal is allowed in the application interview is a critical contingent variable that could determine whether a true test of the proposition is feasible. The skill of the worker, in turn, is a critical intervening variable that can determine the nature of the help given the recipient to find her goal. Including such variables in a research design intended to test the truth of a proposition increases its relevance for practice.

Thus far, the elements involved in formulating a proposition that can guide a principled practice have been noted. Now consider the other side, the commendation element in the principle.

This element must translate ethical imperatives into guides for their realization in action. Whereas the propositional component of a principle usually formulates predictive statements having theoretical relevance, the commendation component authorizes the proposed action. Commendations prescribe the limitations on choice of action open to the worker. Thus, if one envisages the sum of propositional statements and their explanations embodied in practice principles as the knowledge core of the professional practice, the analogous professional values derive from the sum of ethical imperatives sponsoring the commendations included in these same principles.

Principles thus direct the practitioner to the particular task, more sharply focus her awareness upon the practice situation, and most important, integrate purpose and process into a single justification of her conduct. I noted earlier how principles are elaborated in rules that give specific direction to and assure some regularity in prescribed behavior. It is apparent that the order informing the structure and form of the work directed by such rules comes closest to representing the guiding principles incorporated in its production. Although the individual style of the worker and the unique attributes of the recipient lend distinctive features to the product, rarely will they significantly alter its principle-determined structure.

For these various reasons, the practice principle is the most powerful intellectual tool in a profession's practice.

Principles: From Thought to Action

A principle-seeking question asks for guidance in a situation involving uncertainty about values, about knowledge, or about both. For example, suppose a worker visits the home of a terminally ill patient who tells her that he intends to commit suicide and suggests by his manner and tone that he has both the will and the ability to act on his intention. In this situation, the worker confronts an ethical dilemma; and some readily available rule might clarify the appropriate actions. Is it the patient's right, if he so wishes, to terminate his life? Lacking a rule, the worker will search her memory for some guiding principles that might help her generate a rule governing the occasion. She may recall this admonition, "When a patient threatens suicide, the worker should treat the threat as real, unless she has ample reason for thinking otherwise." This practice principle tells her what to do. Pursuing her knowledge and value concerns further, she may seek to recall theories about suicidal patients who are terminally ill and approaches to ethical dilemmas that have addressed similar situations. By now, of course, it should be obvious that the trigger response a rule releases is missing here. Doubts have inhibited action and choice. The worker needs time to think before she acts. Clearly the principle-seeking question differs from rule-seeking questions in that it lacks distinctive indicators that index it for rapid recovery from memory. In this situation, there are no stored rule analogs. In these circumstances, efforts at rule recovery from memory yield no appropriate directive or command. The worker's task now requires her to identify a new class of compositions, to which the one embodied in the principle question would be analogous, and to abstract key indicators that permit the assignment of similar future compositions to this new class. This is obviously a more time consuming and complex mental undertaking than recovering a rule from memory.

Whenever an appeal to principle is required, however, the question that formulates it is characterized by certain necessary elements. This question *must* contain both those variables whose hypothetical relationships are to be defined and the behavioral alternatives from among which a commendable choice must be found. If these elements cannot be identified and included in the question, the question is not likely to be associated with a stored analog indexed to an appropriate principle. If such an association cannot be made, the doubt that inhibits action will persist; and recovery from memory will find only theoretical and ethical imperatives. This shift in turn will direct attention to the context of practice and lead to an attempt to redefine the situation in a way that reopens the path to action.

An appeal to practice principles assumes that some justification for practice can be found within the program and services of the agency. When principles cannot be found, both the program and its services are placed in doubt. Because uncertainty at this level raises questions about the agency, its goals and objectives, and its methods and practice, it understandably cannot long be tolerated. Either a redefinition of function, of eligibility, or of scope — justified by theory and ethical preferences — will be attempted, or service must ultimately cease.

Examples of major programmatic changes resulting from changes in the principles that justify them are readily available. Some historically significant instances include dropping the relief-giving function from voluntary family agencies during the Depression and the institution of the work-relief programs associated with the CCC camps and WPA in the same period.

The prevalence of rules and principles in the literature of practice testifies to the importance attached to both by those best informed about the work to be done. A systematic organization of rules and principles in relation to the elements of work is not readily available, however; and whereas propositions from the behavioral sciences and from practice experience are usually presented as generalizations (without the ethical component that principles require), rules are generally embedded in bureaucratic directives (without reference to the principles that justify them).[13] The elements of work clearly offer a useful framework for the systematizaton of principles and rules. At the most general level, the principles guiding action in relation to unmet needs, to programs and methods, and to procedures for assessing needs in relation to interventive possibilities comprise the wider parameters of social work practice. At a more restricted level, the principles governing policies and procedures, functions and roles, and methods and techniques offer immediately useful guidance in the provision of services. Altogether, such a body of principles organized around the elements of work would offer the profession the means for judging the degree to which any social work practice is justified by principles.

It is useful to note that not all rules are justified by concurrently accepted principles and that not all principles are based on theoretically consistent propositions and ethical imperatives. When they are, the basis for a professional practice is present. This will become more evident as I consider the place of theory and ethics in the practice of social workers.

---

13. See, for example, Jack Rothman, *Planning and Organizing for Social Change: Action Principles from Social Science Research* (New York: Columbia University Press, 1974).

CHAPTER FOUR

»» ««

Theory

EVERY PRACTITIONER should know that her observations are not simply casual scannings; they involve a conceptually ordered search for evidence. Her eyes and ears are trained to help her select evidence relative to some framework that will permit inferences to be drawn, order revealed, meanings surmised, and an explanatory guide for action planned. These organizing frameworks are theories. They provide the conceptual models that help the worker grasp the meaning of the relationships among phenomena that practice leads her to observe.[1]

For example, in seeking to help residents of a low-income housing project avoid eviction because of their poor housekeeping practices, we observed an interesting phenomenon—known to the residents themselves, but frequently denied by management.[2] The household conditions of families that kept up very similar poor housekeeping practices were nevertheless judged differently by housing-staff evaluators. Some were recommended for eviction, while others were not. In an

1. For discussions of frameworks in social work, see *Social Work* 22, no. 5 (September 1977); ibid. 26, no. 1 (January 1981).
2. Harold Lewis and Mildred Guinessy, *Helping the Poor Housekeeping Family in Public Housing: Research and Demonstration Project* (Philadelphia: Friends Neighborhood Guild, 1964).

effort to understand this differential treatment, we studied both categories of families and arrived at a theoretical framework that consistently accounted for the different evaluations. Families that attributed their poor housekeeping to their own failings were not recommended for eviction; families that attributed their poor housekeeping to shortcomings in the management or to other circumstances for which they would accept no responsibility were reported for eviction. We observed further that families who blamed themselves appeared to be *neglectful*—their poor performance was as much a product of omission as it was of commission. Families who blamed the outside world appeared to be *abusive* housekeepers. It was not surprising to note that the management evaluators felt that the neglectful families were likely to do something about their poor practices while the latter families, who were as abusive to the staff as they were to their residences, were unlikely to change their behavior. It thus became evident to us that the judgment to evict was more likely to be based on the evaluator's belief in the possibility of change than it was on the current condition of the housekeeping. We accordingly developed a theoretical framework that typed families as neglectful or abusive and suggested different approaches to helping them improve their housekeeping. In a broader application, this framework seemed useful in situations in which intervention by unwelcome authority is required to correct socially unacceptable practice—in protective services for children, for example, or in police work with juveniles.

Theories are a rich source of propositional statements that inform practice principles. They suggest 'if–then' and 'from this in time to that,' relationships that can help practitioners in their conceptually ordered search for evidence and for guides to action. In our housekeeping study, for example, a causal proposition suggested by the framework might be this: If the client is an abusive housekeeper, the family is likely to be recommended for eviction. A process proposition might be this: In time, the abusive housekeeper's attitude toward the management evaluator will convince him that no change in behavior can be expected, given the intense anger and denial evident; and the evaluator will recommend eviction.

Many practice principles are formulated from experience rather than theory. Nevertheless, such propositions ultimately tend either to be subsumed within a theoretical framework or to be identified as idiosyncratic to agency or worker styles.

An appropriate perspective on the place of practice theory in the work of social workers requires a preliminary consideration of the process whereby professional judgments are made and the manner in which inner-directed questions provide the basis for such judgments.[3] This is so because theory primarily involves intellectual work—work that entails abstraction and conceptualization. Theoretical work is initiated in response to inquiry. It is intended to frame meaningful questions and to provide plausable explanations. To understand the place of theory in practice, it is essential to appreciate how professional questions are shaped by theory and in turn utilize it when the directions needed to guide action are being recovered from memory.

THE PROFESSIONAL QUESTION

THE SOCIAL WORKER in practice must exercise judgments in uncertain situations that are often transient in nature and emotionally trying. Confronted with a variety of observa-

3. For various views of practice theory, see Genevieve W. Carter, "Theory Development in Social Work Research," *Social Service Review* 29, no. 1 (March 1955): 34–42; Bernice Simon, *Relationship between Theory and Practice in Social Casework* (New York: National Association of Social Workers, 1960); Max Siporin, *Introduction to Social Work Practice* (New York: Macmillan Co., 1975), pp. 118–30; Martin Bloom, *The Paradox of Helping* (New York: John Wiley & Sons, 1975), pp. 53–67.

tions, she must integrate what she perceives into a balanced, coherent, and concise composition. Such compositions organize the practice situation for the worker, carry in their design the imprint of her personal style, and manifest in their form the shape of their particular content. A set of such compositions encompasses the worker's comprehension of the circumstances that require her action, suggesting questions whose answers must be recalled from memory. These questions thus provide the worker with the key to her stored knowledge and values, bringing them to bear upon the present situation, defining the range of available choices, as well as their possible consequences, and clarifying the 'givens' to be taken as certainties in an otherwise indeterminate situation.

It may be that all helping situations are inherently uncertain, or it may be that the professional helper and the person seeking help must perceive such situations as uncertain; either or both are possible. Nevertheless, the doubt centers upon the indeterminate elements in the situation, those which cannot be explained by what is already known and valued. In addition to anticipated choices, this uncertainty assures that there are possibilities for finding choices not previously identified. Such choices, stemming from the practice encounter itself, impart to each professional act consequences that further inform the profession and extend the meanings that attach to its values.

Formulating professional questions in uncertain situations can be intellectually demanding and emotionally stressful. The tensions that accompany suspended judgments under circumstances requiring action may be first relieved by the certainties assumed and second brought into focus by their relation to areas of doubt. To be pitilessly simple, both worker and recipient, when both are equally in doubt, can tolerate the uncertainties so long as they do not have to do something, especially when they do not know what to do. The participants in the helping act do not need to identify suspended action with imposed inaction or inhibited action. Both may trust from experience that the unexpected and unexplainable are not uncommon and that time may yield new alternatives and offer better possible choices.[4] Nevertheless, the unknown and the doubt associated with the unknown motivate the professional question and provide the psychic energies needed to set in motion and sustain the recovery effort.

Recovering for use what has been stored in memory is a complex process, incompletely understood. What one remembers is influenced by the associations that have sustained it in mind and by the associations that bring it to recall. What is recovered, therefore, is not be simply what was originally stored. We can assume that when she draws on memory the worker initially stores compositions rather than information bits and that such compositions are altered in the process of storage and recall. It should thus be clear that a professional question delves into memory looking for a contextual analog of images, not for isolated units whose total meaning must then be computed.[5]

It is not clear how what is known and valued is stored in memory. For our purposes, it may be sufficient to assume that the stored compositions are associated in some manner with relevant theory (models), ethical imperatives, princi-

4. Amelie O. Rorty (Discussions among fellows, Center for Advanced Studies in the Behavioral Sciences, Stanford, California, 1970). I am indebted to Professor Rorty for suggestions of ways in which doubts can be sustained in uncertain situations.

5. Robert J. Sternberg, *Intelligence, Information Processing and Analogical Reasoning: The Componential Analysis of Human Abilities* (New York: John Wiley & Sons, 1977), pp. 99–172; David E. Meyer and Robert W. Schranveidt, "Meaning, Memory Structure and Mental Processes," *Science* 192, no. 2 (April 1976): 27-33; Gale Goldberg and Ruth R. Middleman, "Visual Teaching," mimeographed (Louisville, Kentucky: University of Louisville, Kent School of Social Work, n.d.), pp. 2–7.

ples, and rules. New observations enter as compositions and tap their analogs in storage, recovering those directives for practice associated with them. What sustains the recall effort, however, is the desire to reduce tension through action, and what will be crucial to the worker are the actions her knowledge and values suggest. As I pointed out in Chapter 3, rules that command are most likely to offer the quickest access to action directives. Theories and imperatives may color a worker's perspective; but in a moment of decision they are more likely to enter the analog as sources of doubt, inhibiting rather than facilitating action.[6]

Everybody asks questions. Knowledgeable questions are informed by established facts and shaped by current personal and fashionable styles. What is known, as it is embedded in a question, orders, describes, classifies, predicts, and tests. The style that shapes the question arranges, colors, distributes, blends, and balances. Together, the known and the style jointly design the question; but rarely, if ever, are their influences fully manifest in a particular question.[7]

Professional questioning is an understandable tool with which to generate a process of discovery and recovery. Although an isolated professional question may identify moments in this process, the process—not the isolated question—is invested with purpose by the value that directs its elaboration. A pro-

6. Scott Buchanan, *The Doctrine of Signatures: A Defense of Theory in Medicine* (London: Kegan, Paul, Trench, Truboner & Co., 1938); Donald A. Norman, *Memory and Attention* (New York: John Wiley & Sons, 1969); Konrad Z. Lorenz, "Innate Bases of Learning," in *On the Biology of Learning,* ed. Karl A. Pribrian (New York: Harcourt, Brace & World, 1967), pp. 13–93; H.W. Magrum, "Advances in Brain Research with Implications for Learning," ibid., pp. 171–90.

7. R.M. MacIver, "The Modes of the Question Why," *Journal of Social Philosophy* 5 (October 1939–July 1940): 197–205; Noel D. Belnap, Jr., *An Analysis of Questions: Preliminary Report* (Santa Monica, Calif.: Systems Development Corp., 1963).

ductive questioning process thus deliberately seeks to penetrate to the heart of the matter.

Because persons differ in the ways they compose their observations, in what they have available for recall, and in their talent for ferreting out the extraordinary in an otherwise ordinary situation, it is probable that each also develops a personal questioning style. This style may provide the unique attributes of a worker's activity as it combines with the prevalent professional and agency styles that characterize practice.[8]

It is thought that the questioning intent differs among professions. Some professions are worker-centered, with the subject playing the role of informant. In a journalist's questions, for example, the order, timing, range, depth, and direction of the interview primarily serve the information-seeking needs of the questioner, while the informant's needs, goals, and purposes are considered only as they may influence what is to be gained or lost through the inquiry. Other professions are thought to be client-centered. In many branches of psychotherapy, the client's situation, needs, goals, and purposes set the conditions of the process. It is difficult to attribute either of these extremes to any profession, for all probably share both to some extent.

Certainly, the human service professions that attempt to effect changes in the inner and outer environments of client systems must seek the benefits of both approaches to assure a more workable and individually appropriate utilization of this professional tool. In fact, experience suggests that most professional helpers employ both approaches in a single professional encounter. The professional question addressed in this book refers only to the product of a process in which the worker composes her sense impressions and arranges them so as to

8. Harold Lewis, "The Significance for Social Work Education of the Student's Approach to the Formulation of a Research Question," *Social Work Education Reporter* 9, no. 2 (April 1961).

permit effective storage of what is currently evident and to assist effective recovery of the directives to be applied in practice.

This is the query the worker puts to herself, not the question she puts to the recipient. That latter question is used by the worker as a means to obtain material to compose her self-directed question. It would be an error to assume that the worker's data, which provide the substantive material she needs to compose such self-directed questions, are limited to verbal statements. Professional persons assemble data not only through selective sight, touch, taste, and smell, but also through focused listening. Although the worker may silently formulate a sentence that sharply states her inner-directed questions, she is likely to include information derived from all her senses in her composition, in order to appropriately depict her awareness.

Much of the discussion of questioning in the literature is concerned with oral exchange between two or more persons, not with the internal exchanges considered here. Granted the possibility that all interrogational exchanges share many characteristics, differences must be noted.

When the questioner is the person who is also answering the question, the exchange is not a dialogue. Under these circumstances the questioner is not seeking to clarify the meaning of a respondent whose ability, willingness, and opportunity to share what her answer intends may be limited. Nor does the self-respondent have to guess at the range of possible answers implicit in the question. The innermost thoughts and feelings of the questioner are available to the respondent. The exchange, moreover, is bound to be monostylous (and hence congenial), if somewhat slanted. Certainly the intellectual and emotional subtleties that accompany the apprehension of heterogenous styles incorporated into other-directed questions will be absent.

In self-directed questions, when the worker is off base, she is unlikely to discover this fact unless she has internalized cueing processes that both sensitize her to such deviations and signal the need for corrective measures. The sequence of question and answer may not follow a temporal order, given the fluxional state of mental and emotional processes and the spatial dimensions of compositions.

The observation that "knowing what counts as an answer is equivalent to knowing the question," has a special meaning in self-directed questions. In such answers, "what counts" may change in the process of composition and may remain uncertain until the composition has entered storage, recovered guiding directives, tested them against the practice demand that initiated the query, and selectively applied those judged appropriate. It is fundamental to an understanding of professional questioning that we appreciate the intention of the questioner: The query must lead from inquiry to action, and the final definition of "what counts" is "what works."

The differences between self-directed and other-directed questions appear to play some role in structuring the professional practice situation; undoubtedly they have important organizational implications for service delivery. For example, if a worker is off-base in her internal interrogatory process, she may not be aware of this aberration. This possibility suggests the need for some colleagial monitoring, not necessarily supervisory or educational in character, but capable of assuring an extrasystemic cueing procedure as a safeguard in situations where such abberations can have immediate and irreversible impact on recipients.

Characteristics of the Professional Question

The practitioner is often required to act more on the basis of her understanding of a situation than on the basis of her knowledge. Although such understanding is informed by what she knows, it also draws upon beliefs, self-evaluations of emotional states, and unconscious awareness.[9] It is thus possible to see that the worker's understanding, however incomplete, can encompass more than she knows, in the sense of truths. It is also important to appreciate the practitioner's need to maximize certainties and minimize doubts, lest the latter so engage her awareness as to paralyze action entirely. This practical requirement differs from the stance of the knowledge developer, who minimizes certainties and maximizes doubts in order to add to what is known and challenge what is thought to be true. The practitioner has always in mind two different but related questions: "What am I to do now?" and "How am I to act in this situation?"

What am I to do now? Questions of this kind may be dealt with in a variety of ways by the response mechanisms of the body, some of which react instantly without the storage of the information communicated in the inquiry while others store knowledge and need time both to achieve storage and to recover information. I am more concerned with the latter, though I must necessarily give some attention to the processes of habituation, so characteristic of situations in which one learns to operate in accordance with rules.

The pervasive nature of "what to do now" questions, which are normal to any living organism whose survival requires that appetites be satisfied, has been intensified as social interactions have escalated and as technological innovations have quickened the pace of human life. Complicated beings complicate their environment; thereby they face the danger of confusion in relation to vital decisions. To assure one's survival in these circumstances, highly developed orienting tools capable of managing both objective and subjective positioning are clearly required. The crucial attribute of an orienting mechanism is a signaling capacity that quickly alerts its owner

9. David Rapaport, *Emotions and Memory*, 2d ed. (New York: International Universities Press, 1950).

both to what is to be avoided and to what is to be preferred in a great variety of circumstances. Such attributes, which are evident in the behavioral directives stemming from the brain and nervous system, are consciously manifest in theories and ethics.

Theory and ethics provide the underpinnings of rational action possible; they are possibly the most developed rational programs that persons have for orienting themselves to their environment. This assertion requires further amplification.

In professional questioning, the "what to do now" question is composed within the context of natural, man-made, and interpersonal processes. In their form, content, and relationships, they convey an orienting perspective, and they suggest the range of acceptable value choices in the given circumstances. The location of the professional encounter, its timing and duration, the furnishings of its setting, the dress and manner of its participants, and its formal or informal personal contacts (with their accompanying rhetoric) convey as much of what the agency values as do the conditions of eligibility, including the process whereby these conditions are ascertained. These artifacts and interpersonal processes orient the worker to norms of an agency's program and service and define for her the range of outcomes likely to fall within the scope of its objectives and goals. In practice, these artifacts and personal contacts are omnipresent, providing persistent and consistent reenforcement for the worker's perspective. They incorporate cueing devices that alert her to possible departures from acceptable behavioral norms. Unlike commendations and commands, the imperatives imparted by the atmosphere surrounding the professional encounter permeate everything that occurs within it and point the action in the direction of its purpose. They nevertheless provide no guidance as to how to achieve it.

Theory provides a framework within which the materials to be included in composing the professional question can be assembled. Artifacts and personal contacts are conceptually ordered by theoretical orientations. Unlike imperatives, theories orient the worker to observations that concern means rather than ends. A wide range of differing (sometimes inconsistent) theories can thus be concurrently entertained by a worker. They serve to orient her to different aspects of the professional situation; and each is likely to be most effectively influenced by means dovetailed to its peculiar attributes.[10]

The importance of these assertions that theory and ethics play an orienting role and that they are pervasive in professional encounters lies in their implications for the composition of the professional question. Clearly, such orientation aides provide a regulatory device of a sort and monitor the scope and manner, as well as the content, of observations and evaluations. What they add through economy of effort, however, they may sacrifice by weakening the potential for innovative apprehensions—those that reach beyond the limits of agency and professional purpose and prevalent practice methods.

"What to do now" questions are likely to draw heavily for theory on the human sciences, on relevant service professions, and on the humanities for the variety of forms in which propositional formulations may be manifest. These theories inform about the 'what' and 'why' of practice. The very special function they serve, and the manner in which this purpose requires that they be formulated, limits their usefulness for that part of practice which poses the second question, "How am I to act in this situation?"

How am I to act? Intonation, gesture, inversion of text, special markings, and context cues have been used to signal 'ques-

10. For general analysis, see Marx W. Wartofsky, *Conceptual Foundations of Scientific Thought* (New York: The Macmillan Co., 1968), pp. 240–87; for specific application, Mary Louise Somers, "Four Small Group Theories: A Comparative Analysis and Evaluation of Selected Social Science Theory for Use as Teaching Content in Social Group Work" (D.S.W. diss., Western Reserve University, 1957).

tion' to the brain.[11] These signals solicit responses when those perceiving them assume that an inquiry requiring clarification is intended. Where nothing is in doubt, questions are likely to be treated as positioning statements rather than inquiries.

Where doubt is present, as it inevitably must be in a help-seeking situation, choice becomes relevant and decisions become problematic. The anguish of the recipient whose cry for help conveys her inability to act so as to escape from intolerable circumstances, is not likely to be assuaged by an answer that simply redefines her situation — unless the redefinition itself alters her circumstance.

The professional question generated by the request for help represents something other than the "what am I to do now?" apparently conveyed by the recipient's appeal. Although the recipient seems to be asking for possible alternatives from among which she may choose, the worker understands that the request includes more. If she exercises her professional judgment intelligently, the worker will evaluate the recipient's ability, willingness, and opportunities to make those choices.[12] Her evaluation in fact defines the uncertain professional practice situation confronting the worker. If she seeks guidance through self-directed inquiry, her situation will not be altered unless the response she recovers shows how to proceed with *this* recipient. In the final analysis, 'how to' professional questions must be answered if action is to be taken.

11. I am indebted to Dwight L. Bolinger of Harvard University for discussions of ways in which 'question' may be signaled to the brain (Center for Advanced Study in the Behavioral Sciences, Stanford, California, 1969).

12. See Lillian Ripple, "Motivation, Capacity and Opportunity: Studies in Casework Theory and Practice," *Social Service Monographs,* 2d ser. (Chicago: University of Chicago School of Social Service Administration, 1964), pp. 19–39, for an effort to incorporate these worker evaluations into a practice theory.

For the practitioner, question cues must serve both as sources of information and signals. In the inquiry they promote, they convey the elements to be used in estimating the range of possible choices open to the worker, thus helping her to choose among 'how to' alternatives. In this sense, appropriately composed 'how to' questions convey to the memory the form of what can count as an answer, and recovery from memory offers the possibility of clarifying the uncertainty that inhibits worker action. Such questions seek to recapture an intact directive for action in uncertain situations. The reasoning is analogical.[13] The worker asks herself for an example of a situation similar to the one being confronted, and wills her recall to carry with it an associated action directive. The logical form of these questions demands reasoning by proportions: "This is to this as that is to that." Although the guiding principle or rule then recovered will include or imply the causal (or process) proposition, the utility of the analog lies in the power of the imagery it provides. It allows for a large measure of inference, a quick, succinct assurance of relevance, and some confidence that the action guide may be appropriate to the tasks at hand.

For example, the worker may note the aged applicant dropping into the chair, breathing rapidly in short, deep inhalations, palms sweating and face flushed. She recalls an analogous observation that carries with it the suggestion: "anxiety!! — put the client at ease." The worker may immediately open a line of discussion calculated to reassure the applicant. Of course, should the client remark, "Climbing five flights of stairs because of a bum elevator is exhausting," the worker is likely to revise her assessment on the spot.

Theory points the worker toward, and guides her in the

13. R.V. Davis and L.T. Siojo, "Analytical Reasoning: A Review of the Literature," Technological Report no. 1 (Minneapolis: University of Minnesota Department of Psychiatry, 1972).

selection of, information useful to the composition of professional questions. For the 'how to' question, rule and principle complement this effort. They are more exact and more readily recoverable in a form useful for action because they are associated with analogical processes.

THEORY AS EXPLANATION

THEORY IN SOCIAL WORK is also intended to provide explanations for what happens in practice.[14] These explain why the participants in the service relationship behave the way they do and are what they are. Rules and principles may provide reasons why the social worker does what she does; but they do not in themselves explain the 'why' of her actions. The explanation for this ultimately rests with the theories that justify both the propositions in principles and the directives in rules. Theories impose no conditions on the use of the understanding they communicate — an essential attribute of rules and principles.

A theory may be taken to mean more than the generalizations it embodies. As noted earlier, in social work literature, theory is often thought to provide a model of the phenomena that generalizations describe and to fill a heuristic function while serving as an aid to understanding. No systematic theoretical model that attempts to explain all of social work practice has thus far been proposed, but many ad hoc models of a more limited nature have been entertained. Social work has

14. E. Madden, "The Nature of Psychological Explanation," *Methods* 9 (1957): 53–63; R. B. Braithwaite, *Scientific Explanation* (Cambridge: At the University Press, 1955); Alan Ross Anderson and O.K. Moore, "Models in the Social Sciences," in *Concepts, Theory and Explanation in Behavioral Science*, ed. Gordon J. Direnzo (New York: Random House, 1966), pp. 75–92.

also utilized nontheoretical models to depict the drama of practice.[15] Such models order their constituents so as to suggest their role and place in practice, but they offer no explanations of either. They are not to be confused with theoretical models, which order their variables in a way that suggests propositions to be tested.

Simple recognition of the wide range of phenomena that concern social workers cautions against any attempt to arrive at a single comprehensive practice theory. Instead, efforts have concentrated on developing generalizations from practice and incorporating formulations developed in the human sciences and service professions into social work practice. Such efforts contribute to the practice science of social work, which must be based on propositions derived from principles of practice and confirmed by evidence meeting acceptable standards of credibility.

The scientific disciplines generally tend to partition knowledge about man and the environment with which he interacts into discrete segments. For social work, such a partitioning merely serves to fragment the knowledge needed for practice. Knowledge of persons, of their biosocial functioning, and of the societal context in which they experience their time in the cosmos must be synthesized to achieve its greatest usefulness for professions fulfilling identifiable social purposes. Indeed, social work constructs much of its view of practice on the basis of such synthesized knowledge.

Characteristically, such knowledge is formulated as knowledge of 'what' and 'what for'; but as noted earlier, it must be supplemented by knowledge of 'how to.' For example, in a model of practice that uses the impromptu drama as its analog (i.e., functional social work), agency, recipient,

15. For example, Harold Lewis, "The Functional Approach to Social Work Practice: A Restatement of Assumptions and Principles," *Journal of Social Work Process* 15 (1966): 115–34.

worker, need, and resource each plays a special role in the process of providing service. The following generalizations (not necessarily confirmed truths) about each of these elements of the model are useful assumptions in an approach to practice. Clearly, they are not based on evidence drawn exclusively from social work practice — they utilize observations from the full range of human experience.[16]

Agency:

(what) Social agencies are institutional expressions of the community's concern for its collective well-being.

(what for) Community resources from public and private sources are allocated to social agencies to meet the welfare needs of its citizens.

Recipient:

(what) The recipient has the potential for discovering solutions to his problems, but he may need help in realizing this potential.

(what for) A recipient's condition and the need that condition is judged to reflect provide the basis for community concern and the ultimate justification for allocating community resources.

Worker:

(what) The worker is an agent of that part of the community that has sanctioned and provided the resource.

(what for) The worker is expected to provide a psychological climate that facilitates the formation and maintenance of the worker-recipient relationship through which service is provided.

16. Ibid., pp. 123–31.

Need:

> (what) Conditions that must be dealt with for the community's well-being constitute the unmet needs for which the services of social agencies are intended.
>
> (what for) Conditions for which services are intended lay legitimate claims on community resources, within the limits set by community norms, to the extent that a recipient's expressed needs are viewed as needs that can be met by the services of an agency.

Resource:

> (what) At any time, identifiable human needs in a community will appear to exceed the resources available to meet them.
>
> (what for) Agency resources carry inherent limitations affecting the uses to which they can be put; and together with recipient need, they represent the social component in the service relationship.

Service:

> (what) Service is the incorporated community resource created in the worker–recipient transaction as a tangible agency program unit.
>
> (what for) Service as a concrete social resource carries the potential for material help (i.e., meeting of need). Service as an expression of the way in which resources are provided carries the potential for psychological help.

Such generalizations are necessary in formulating a theory of practice. Expanding their scope, adding generalizations of a similar order, and establishing their truth with increased rigor, however, will not provide explanations of the 'how to' type essential to a complete practice science. Statements about the nature of man, the human condition, the social milieu, institutional organization, agency structure, needs, resources, and service abound in social work literature. What is known about each of these subjects constitutes a body of knowledge of substantial scope, constantly undergoing reformulation in the human sciences and service professions. Service professions, however, are concerned with using this necessary knowledge in administering services in a helpful way. Through the development of knowledge gained in the process of providing such help, practice makes its distinctive contributions to all of human knowledge. Although a practice science utilizes the 'what' and 'what for' types of knowledge, it must systematically relate such knowledge to 'how to' statements in order to explain itself. Principles of practice incorporate such generalizations, thus providing practice science with its unique knowledge attributes.

The relationship between social work practice and the human sciences described here is not unlike that described by Herbert A. Simon when he asserts that professions need a science of design (i.e., practice science) which incorporates theories that explain the design process. Simon notes that, "Everyone designs who devises courses of action aimed at changing existing situations into preferred ones. . . . Design, so construed, is the core of all professional training; it is the principal mark that distinguishes the professions from the sciences."[17] Simon argues that natural science impinges on an artifact (goal-setting system) through two of the three terms of the relation that characterizes it: the structure of the artifact itself and the environment in which it performs.[18] The human sciences impinge on social work in an analogous fashion. For social work, the two terms would be the context of practice and the human resource elements involved in its

17. Herbert A. Simon, *The Sciences of the Artificial* (Cambridge: MIT Press, 1969), p. 55.
18. Ibid., p. 6.

performance. The third term in Simon's scheme is the point of convergence between the inner and outer environments, the artifact itself, which is analogous to the professional helping process in social work practice. Simon seeks theories concerning the 'how to' of practice not encompassed by 'what' or 'what for' statements. Simon's formulations reflect the continued interest of all professions in the possibility of a practice science.

Social work formulations about practice tend to be definition oriented and to draw primarily on descriptive studies for their evidence. Theories that represent interrelated definitions and hypotheses (the latter verified by studies that test their truth or falsehood) are rare.

Most frequently, a proposed approach to practice is composed of a set of interrelated definitions but no hypotheses.[19] The approaches to practice encompassed in 'diagnostic' and 'functional' social work, for example, were of this order. Efforts to elicit explanations of practice through means other than hypothesis testing have produced formulations that principally serve classificatory purposes—attempts, for example, to reconceptualize practice in terms of game theory, systems theory, role theory, or the like. These formulations are more appropriately described as alternate frames of reference.

Whenever practice theories in social work have attempted to incorporate tested hypotheses in their formulations, they have been restrictive in scope. It is probable that an inclusive theory will not become possible until many such more limited formulations upon which to build have been developed.[20] It is unlikely that social work practice will move

19. Hans L. Zattenberg, *On Theory and Verification in Sociology* (New York: Tressler Press, 1954).

20. Theodore N. Ferdinand, "On the Impossibility of a Complete, General Theory of Behavior," *The American Sociologist* 414 (November 1969); 30–32.

significantly beyond definition and classification formulations so long as the studies used for verification of hypotheses are primarily descriptive.

» »   « «

The directive side of rules and principles, which links action to theory, must be matched with the command and commendations that give them purpose if both the means and the ends of practice are to be jointly understood. For this reason, it is useful to consider the place of ethics in a practice science as the other side of the principles that guide its actions.

CHAPTER FIVE

»»   ««

Ethics

ETHICAL IMPERATIVES are useful intellectual tools for professional practitioners. The prescriptive commands contained in moral principles constitute the core of professional codes of ethics.[1] Such codes are among the more important statements inductees are encouraged to read and follow. Professions believe that practice should be moral; and to assure a moral practice, guidance needs to be provided to the practitioner.

The power of this tool lies in its specification of what the practitioner must, should, or ought to do in order that values affirmed by the profession be realized in practice. Because it is often unclear how the ethical imperative is realized in a principled practice, the initial section of this chapter considers the need for this tool and attempts to clarify the process whereby it is put to use. Also of interest to a profession is the manner in which an ethical imperative is formulated.

---

1. For a brief discussion of the function of a code of ethics and a systematic effort to develop such a code, see "Revising the U.S. Senate Code of Ethics," *Hastings Center Report* 11, no. 1 (February 1981): Special Supplement pp. 1–28; see also Charles W. McCann, "The Code of Ethics of the N.A.S.W.: An Inquiry into Its Problems and Perspectives," in *Values in Social Work Education,* ed. Boyd E. Olvatt (Salt Lake City: University of Utah Graduate School of Social Work, 1977), pp. 10–19.

The second section attempts to satisfy this interest by providing illustrative examples of attempts to formulate ethical imperatives for social work practice.

THE NEED FOR
ETHICAL IMPERATIVES

THE ACTIONS OF THE WORKER, from which one can infer the morality that informs her practice, provide the ultimate test of adherence to professional values. Moral maturity in a helping relation is recognized in all human service professions as a necessary prerequisite to achieving an important psychological influence in the service transaction.[2]

Workers talk seriously about shared standards, rights, and obligations — contractual arrangements involving mutual agreement and expectations of positive consequences. Undergirding such talk is an assumption about behavior that is based on conscious and universal logical principles and founded on mutual respect and trust.

For good and sound reasons, social workers are concerned to prevent the unwarranted imposition of moral judgments in their relationships with recipients.[13] The history of punitive and discriminatory actions affecting workers and recipients alike reflects negative community attitudes toward dependent people and community misconceptions both about people who seek social work help and about workers who provide such help. As a consequence, most discussions of morality among workers have been concerned with avoiding moral prejudice in the helping relationship. Less consi-

2. Harold Lewis, "Morality and the Politics of Practice," *Social Casework* 53, no. 7 (July 1972): 404–17.

3. Charles S. Levy, *Social Work Ethics* (New York: Human Science Press, 1976), pp. 55–78.

deration has been given to the ethical behavior that should shape their practice.[4]

Workers do not intend their practice to be devoid of standards that assure morally mature behavior. They realize the need for honest, trusting, fair behavior, and they become critical when they observe evidence of its absence. They decry abusive, manipulative, devious actions and deplore such behavior as unprofessional — by which they mean unethical. In reacting to what they believe to be immoral behavior, they are in effect assuming their profession's commitment to a set of values.

Work understandably directs the worker's attention to the effects of her efforts rather than the values such effects are intended to uphold. Restrictions on choices available to both recipient and worker, for example, are typically perceived as problems to be solved rather than unwarranted intrusions on freedom. Inequities in the distribution of resources are rationalized as compromises dictated by what is available and sought rather than by-products of a planned, unfair system of distributive justice. Impediments that stifle trust in the helping relationship are viewed either as defensive ploys used by troubled personalities or as pragmatic responses of hard-pressed agencies seeking to husband limited resources. Rarely are they regarded as expressions of the pervasive societal disregard of fraternal concern, of which such distrust is but one manifestation.[5]

Workers want to believe that their work promotes a moral practice. For example, in seeking to overcome the observed re-

4. A significant exception to this statement can be seen in the extensive effort from 1977 to 1980 devoted to revising the National Association of Social Workers Code of Ethics, under the leadership of Charles Levy.

5. Harold Lewis, "Informal Support Networks and the Welfare State: Some Ethical Considerations," in *Community Support Systems and Mental Health: Research, Practice and Policy,* ed. David E. Biegel and Arthur J. Naparstek (New York: Springer Publishing Co., 1982).

straints that hinder the provision of service, they are driven to learn as much as can be known about such restraints. This knowledge and the reasoning required to attain it makes it possible for workers to consider new approaches to their practice and to enhance the opportunities for worker and recipient alike to choose from among a larger set of relevant alternatives.[6]

The choices a worker must make inevitably reflect her preferences. For example, although she may believe that all persons are to be treated as equals, she may also realize that equality by no means assures equity. Any worker who regularly experiences either the unequal consequences of equal units of service or the unequal utilization of resources that accompanies services claiming to provide equal access will be sensitive to this distinction. Her sensitivity often does not extend to an appreciation of the priority placed on equity by the disadvantaged recipient and on equality by the advantaged. The former seeks distributive justice while the latter hopes to maintain the relative advantages he is free to enjoy under the prevailing conditions of service. Workers frequently must be content to provide recipients with the resources their agencies and they themselves can afford, which may be less than the recipient needs, particularly the most disadvantaged. Workers are not unaware of the inequities in programs that offer more choices to some than they do to others despite the similarity of documented needs. Of the two, equality and equity, the worker often will find it easier to give precedence to equality while deploring the inequities such equality helps sustain.

In her day-to-day work, the worker may not see existing service inequities as evidence of a general failure to assure social justice. She is more likely to be concerned lest the recipient in need be denied access to a particular service from which she can benefit. Solutions to such access problems may

6. Levy, *Social Work Ethics,* pp. 117–20.

take the form of deliberate decisions to allocate a portion of a resource at reduced cost to the recipient or of service schedules organized to lessen the burden on those who have greatest difficulty in managing time or of programs that give priority to the disadvantaged. The equity problem is reduced to a simple problem of policy and procedure affecting intake, eligibility, or some other function. Rarely will the worker feel compelled to address the broad societal influences that contribute to this serious injustice. The worker's actions may appear to contribute to an ethically just practice, even when this very practice implicates the society that sponsors it in a universal injustice.

It would be helpful if the worker could draw upon codified experience in confronting situations that require ethical judgments of the type described.[7] It is both unsettling and time consuming to decide each instance as though, in all respects, it posed a unique moral choice. Practice principles, of course, are intended to provide such codified wisdom, and the commendations contained in them impart the ethical endorsement the worker needs.

FROM ETHICS TO ACTION: THE PROCESS

COMMENDATIONS, AS NOTED EARLIER, are justified by appeals to ethical imperatives. The imperative prescribes the behavior required to achieve a moral practice consistent with claimed values. When a practice principle commands a

7. Dr. Charles W. McCann, a member of the Professional Standards Cabinet and chairperson of the National Committee on Inquiry, N.A.S.W., summarizes his experiences as follows: "[The] Code of Ethics is incomplete. Its deficiencies center in its high level of abstraction and lack of practice utility." McCann, "Code of Ethics," p. 18.

worker to carry out some action, this command contains moral authority because it is endorsed by an ethical imperative. In effect, the principle states that if you do as I say, you can expect to achieve what I predict, and you *should* do what I say since what I advise is both true and right.

For example, a practice principle might state, "Clients shall participate in decisions that affect them." Confronted with a choice in an actual service encounter, a worker can draw on this principle for guidance. The principle informs her that if clients participate in decisions that affect them they are more likely to act on those decisions than they would be if they did not participate. The "shall" element links the principle to its ethical justification.

This mental process has implications for all practice. If it accurately reflects what happens when a worker faces ethical choices, she cannot operate on the basis of practice principles and concurrently engage in unethical practice. Moreover, since professional interventions are intentional and since their consequences are expected to achieve preferred ends, they are never free of moral choices.[8] The ethical dimension, not the theory of the action, provides assurance to the worker that what can be done *ought* to be done.

Process Overview

I am suggesting that there is a process, however imperfectly understood, whereby principled behavior is achieved. The individual worker needs to determine for herself that the propositions and ethical commendations of the principles are both true and right in a moral sense; and to make this determination she must usually experience in practice the consequences that follow from their application. In relation to the

8. C.I. Lewis, *An Analysis of Knowledge and Valuation* (LaSalle, Ill.: Open Court, 1946, reprinted 1962).

principles proposed, she may find personal and social reasons for supporting their directives because she recognizes that they are intended to increase the choices open to recipients. As she works with recipients and discovers for herself the ways in which personal and social factors contribute to the conditions she seeks to change, she will compose the self-confirming proofs that develop and sustain convictions for storage in memory, and she will become more willing to act upon them.

One cannot legislate an inner-directed adherence to an ethic or to truth, but one can promote a context that encourages such adherence. A practice environment that is increasingly intolerant of workers who profess ideals but fail to evidence conviction about them in their work is likely to inspire principled behavior. This fact is sensed by workers who seek employment in agencies where they assume they will be encouraged to follow ethical principles. The social work profession not only attaches considerable importance to its code of ethics but also seeks a sympathetic community environment that encourages the profession to act on the basis of its convictions.

The profession is aware of its limited capacities and of its deficiencies in skill, but there is likewise much evidence of community restraints and deprivations harmful to programs that employ social workers and tending severely to limit these workers' opportunities to achieve at the level of their known capacities.

A measure of a practitioner's skill is her ability to assimilate both the recipient situation and her own situation so as to develop a balanced perspective that frees her to act on the basis of practice principles. In developing and sustaining a conviction to act on these principles, the practitioner must experience work and the opportunity to observe the consequence of her work. An assumption long held by social work educators — that methods are mastered in their application — rests in part on this necessity to do in order to know what it really means to act in a principled way.

Besides clarifying the process whereby a worker-held value is imparted to practice, this perspective also highlights the hierarchical arrangement that helps shape this process. In seeking to operationalize values, ethical imperatives move the general, abstract formulation of preferences to a prescriptive level; and for this reason, the linkage of the imperative to the value is direct. Without such a direct linkage, the imperative can hardly be justified by its requirement that workers adhere to it. In turn, the behavior and attitudes commended by practice principles—expressed in terms of what one ought, must, will, or shall do in certain situations—is hardly likely to inspire adherence in the absence of ethical justifications. Thus commendations are directly linked to imperatives, and through them to values. Finally, the command side of rule-governed behavior draws its authority from the commended actions implicit in principles. This assures a direct linkage from command to commendation to imperative to value. Given this hierarchical, pyramid-like structure, each level embedded in the next and all in the same basic value, it is clear why changes in values and imperatives occur very slowly. Compared to the rapidity of changes in the knowledge base, a change in basic value is like the tortoise to the hare.

This perspective also helps to clarify the assertion so frequently made in the professional literature that all practice is value based. This perspective suggests, moreover, why it cannot be otherwise without sacrificing the purposes that justify professional interventions.

FORMULATING ETHICAL IMPERATIVES

WHETHER WE ACCEPT the description of the process proposed or prefer another, there remains the need for ethical imperatives. How are such imperatives developed?

Starting with Individual Case Situations

One approach would be inductive, deriving a general guiding imperative from lessons learned in individual cases. How this may occur is best demonstrated by an illustrative case.

Consider this situation confronting a group of social workers, in which the need for ethical prescriptions to guide their choices is glaringly evident. In a large city, these social workers testified in private before an N.A.S.W. chapter committee to instances of discriminatory practice against minority children which they had observed in their own or related social service organizations.[9] Partly on the basis of their testimony, the N.A.S.W. chapter entered an amicus brief in a court case charging such discrimination. Lawyers for the plaintiffs asked the chapter to solicit testimony from social workers because they needed specific instances to develop their case. None of those who appeared to testify in private were willing to step forward to do so in public. Fear of reprisal appeared to be the major, albeit not the only reason for their reluctance. They were also concerned about the confidentiality owed both to their clients and to the agency that employed them. What guidance could be given these workers if their actions are intended to support those values that can contribute to morally mature professional behavior?

At the very least, one expects the truth will be told. Although courage will clearly be required to face any threat of retribution for uttering the truth, we are not concerned with courage—an instrumental value—at this point. Ideally, the worker should be free from any constraints that might hinder the reporting of the truth; and both recipient and agency should likewise be secure in knowing that the truth and nothing but the truth will in the short and long runs prove most beneficial for all concerned. To tell the truth,

9. "Professional Ethics and the Wilder versus Sugarman Suit," *Currents* (Newsletter of the New York City Chapter, N.A.S.W.), July 1975.

however, one must trust; and without trust there is no expectation that truth will help. Trust, in practice an essential condition for respect and interdependence, is one ingredient that appears to be in short supply.

The truth is often complex, however, not simple. In addition to the belief that what is asserted is so, there must also be evidence and rules of evidence to demonstrate that what is believed is in fact true. Finally, instances must be available of the claimed truth, or the entire rationale is reduced to a mental exercise of little moment for the case at hand. Thus, to know the truth implies more than a minor form of knowing, and to base action on securely established knowledge requires freedom to consider alternate beliefs, to weigh all the evidence available, to evaluate evidence objectively, to cite examples without undue restraint, in short, to make the choices such freedom permits. Finally, truths do not speak for themselves: They need persons to give voice to their substance. Not all persons are equally able and motivated to speak up, nor do all have the same opportunity. Certainly, in contentious situations there is always a danger that equality will not assure equity and that those more disadvantaged (in this instance the children themselves) may have the least opportunity to vouch for the truth as they perceive it. Trust, choice, and equity must thus be present if in fact a morally mature expression of professional behavior is to be achieved. Ethical issues clearly permeate this case; and how these workers resolve them will seriously affect the results of the ajudication. An ethical imperative that could guide them would obviously be preferred to alternative ways of dealing with the dilemma they face.

Another issue is the question of the right to know as it is manifest in choices affecting medical malpractice insurance. The situation concerns information sharing and the patient's right to be informed in situations where there is conflicting clinical evidence whether it is good for him to know. A physician prescribes a drug for his patient. At issue is the question: how much information should he share with the patient concerning (1) The side-effects that might accompany the beneficial affects of the drug; (2) the success/failure ratio of experimental tests on the drug; and (3) alternative drugs he prefers not to use that claim similar results. Apparently, the extent to which malpractice suits are encouraged because doctors share information of this sort is not clear; but it is of sufficient concern to suggest caution in arriving at a standard for recommended clinical practice. This medical example is also analogous in many respects to the information-sharing dilemmas social workers face in their work.

Denying information to recipients is one of the most controlling forms of knowledge-related behavior in which a worker can participate. Lacking knowledge, recipients are denied the chance to make rational choices and thus denied their freedom. By withholding information, the worker increases her power over the helping relationship: By sharing knowledge she defuses the mystification of professional authority and invites the recipient to share the doubts and uncertainties that are her lot. Because recipients are neither equal in their ability to ferret out the information they want (from worker or elsewhere) nor equally equipped to understand the implications that follow from such information, it is likely that those with the greatest potential access to information will also have the greatest potential for utilizing it. Thus, what and how the worker shares can directly affect the equity of the service.

In the helping relationship, sharing information about self and about elements entering into the relationship is often the most meaningful way trust can be expressed by both parties. For the most disadvantaged recipient, it may be the only way of sharing respect, encouragement, and interdependence. Such personal demonstrations of trust are not to be taken lightly by recipient or worker. How ought the worker behave?

At the very least, one expects that the worker will provide the recipient with any information needed in carrying out a prescribed regimen. The social work code of ethics describes this expectation as "practicing social work within the recognized knowledge and competence of the profession." If this seems to provide a thin veil of protection for the recipient with regard to ethical practice, it nevertheless is the only part of the code that can be liberally interpreted to cover the information-sharing dilemma. But the worker's obligation to prescribe is not the ambiguity at issue; the assumption in this obligation is that the recipient trusts the worker's claim to knowledge and accordingly accepts her authority. At issue is the question of sharing information with the recipient that can open up choices — including possible rejection of the prescription. The freedom this grants the recipient includes risks in which the worker must share, yet all enjoyment of freedom entails risks.

Even more is involved: The sharing of information points up the need for the worker to respect the right of the recipient to choose some risks the worker may not see as warranted. By assisting a recipient to achieve a level of self-trust that supports her risk of independent behavior, the worker demonstrates a willingness to help clarify tasks, monitor behavior, identify weaknesses, and expand on available alternatives. The consequences of her effort are evident to the recipient in his own experience — he is in effect able to know and claim his own growth. He can willingly yield some control to the worker, whose authority is knowingly based on his belief in her capacity to provide the service needed. Her authority is based on means, not ends.

If the recipient chooses to reject the prescription of the worker, however, and the worker seeks to use her professional authority to compel adherence to what she believes to be an appropriate recipient involvement in the service, a different kind of trust is involved. As far as the recipient is concerned, imposition of a choice in these circumstances asks him to trust the worker's intentions rather than her competence; and intentions are never free of the societal constraints that shape them. Thus in the practice situation, the recipient must believe that the policies that govern the practice are just and respectful, that the worker is both fair and friendly, and that the worker places the recipient's interest ahead of all other interests—including the worker's own.[10]

Other questions confront similar issues. For example, what implications for a moral practice flow from a theory of helping that is wholly deterministic, one that assumes that the recipient is not really free to make valid choices?[11] What significant modifications of a democratic ethos occur when a mechanization of service delivery removes the human, caring interface between organization rituals and recipient participation in service?

In confronting these problems in ethics, some generalizations may serve to illustrate the nature of the guiding imperatives to be sought. First, one ought not belittle the efforts, pragmatic and existential, that workers make to assure that reason, justice, and friendship are ingredients in their practice. It is not such efforts, but the implications for ethical practice that flow from failures fully to explore their ethical dimensions, that need more attention.

It appears likely that for some time into the future human service professions will be confronted with a relative dwindling of resources and heightening of program deficiencies. Needs are currently accumulating at a far more rapid rate than our society is becoming willing to meet them. For this reason, it is impor-

10. Harold Lewis, "The Client's Interest," mimeographed (New York: Hunter College School of Social Work, 1980).

11. Alan Keith-Lucas & Elliott, S.A., "Political Theory Implicit in Social Casework Theory," *American Political Science Review* 47, no. 4 (December 1953): 1076–91.

tant to realize that the values implicit in these examples are neither conflicting nor mutually exclusive.

In the helping relationship, societal and practice preferences influence the extent to which reason, justice, and friendship can find expression. Being aware of these influences and their probable consequences, the worker should find it ethically sound in situations where ethical ambiguities make difficult choices more difficult to ask herself these questions:

1. Am I sacrificing the recipient's moral rights in order to assure what I believe is good for him? Am I putting reason before justice? If the answer is yes, I should provide for adequate representation of the recipient's rights by competent counsel.
2. Am I departing from what I know to be good or right for the recipient in order to achieve rapport in the helping situation? Am I putting friendship and caring before reason and justice? If the answer is yes, I must be able to justify such departure with demonstrated achievement of greater well-being and equity for the client. A friendly, encouraging, respectful, and caring relationship is not necessarily a helpful one.[12]

Through such questions, experience is generating an ethical imperative still in its formative stage. To arrive at a firmer guideline, one must locate practice in the wider societal context with which it interacts. One must assume there is a predictable relationship between the two, regardless of the theoretical framework that informs the practice. This relationship is evidenced in the roles of the worker and recipient in the helping process.

12. Harold Lewis, "Values and Ideology in the Profession: Implications in Social Work Practice" (Paper presented at Adelphi University School of Social Work Alumni Conference, Garden City, New York, October 23, 1976).

In times of radical community change when ideologies are in question and programs are in turmoil, both the worker and the recipient see the worker as someone *in* the service of the recipient. In times of expanding resources and reformulation of problems, both see the worker as someone working *with* the recipient in a joint effort to reach shared intentions. In a time of dwindling resources and political and economic conservatism when the worker retreats to the core of her professional claim (her skill in methods), she becomes an expert doing *for* the recipient what is judged to be in his interest. Emphasis on equality, fraternity, and freedom — and their practice counterparts, justice, friendship, and reason — correspond to these role changes and contribute to the formulation of the imperative.

A DEDUCTIVE APPROACH

THUS FAR, OUR DISCUSSION of ethical imperatives suggests the manner in which the worker's actions and the alternatives available to her may generate rules of conduct congenial to her value preferences. An alternate approach to an appreciation of the place of ethical imperatives in shaping a practice is to assume such an imperative and deduce from it the practice principles that would contribute to an ethical performance.

For example, recognizing the importance of distributive justice in the provision of social work services, let us posit an ethical imperative to guide practice decisions in relation to this value.

Recipients of social service programs are among the most disadvantaged in our society. Usually, social workers employed in these programs either serve such recipients directly or work with persons interested in promoting services for them. A moral justification for professional social work practice can therefore be found in the dedication of the practitioner to improving the circumstances and expectations of these recipients. A helping profession not based in some morality that inspires a just order runs the risk of encouraging a practice that promotes an unjust one.

Although by no means the whole of a just order, distributive justice is a particular concern of a helping profession serving the disadvantaged. If professional practice penalizes the least advantaged, it defeats efforts intended to aid the disadvantaged.

An ethical imperative intended to guide the behavior of persons seeking distributive justice has been proposed by John Rawls.[13] Professor Rawls utilizes social contract theory and a set of value expectations that rational persons may be presumed to want (that is, liberty and opportunity, income and wealth, health and educated intelligence, and self-respect) to propose the following necessary conditions for distributive justice:

1. Each person is to have an equal right to the most extensive basic liberty compatible with a similar liberty for others.
2. Social and economic inequalities are to be arranged so that they are both
   (a) reasonably expected to be to everyone's advantage and
   (b) attached to positions and offices equally open to all.

Professor Rawls assumes a framework of social institutions in which equitable and equal opportunity obtains. His second condition suggests an ethical imperative: "The higher expectations of those better situated in the basic structure are just if and only if they work as part of a scheme which improves the expectations of the least advantaged members of society."[14] He also assumes that the first condition must be

13. John Rawls, *A Theory of Justice* (Cambridge: Harvard University Press, Belknap Press, 1971).
14. Ibid., p. 75.

satisfied before the second can be met. Thus the principle of the equal right to liberty becomes a precondition to the establishment of justifiable inequalities. These conditions and the derived ethical imperatives seem compatible with the goals voiced in the literature of social work and in statements expressing program intentions of social services.

Social institutions incorporate in their practice those established patterns of behavior they are charged to maintain in the society that supports them. Although they may differ in their functions in relation to the status quo—some primarily concerned with control or maintenance, others with the restoration or restructuring of social relationships among competing groups—all are directly involved in activities or events that inevitably favor some and may discriminate against others.

Using knowledge of the role of social institutions in any society and applying the ethical imperative earlier enunciated for achieving distributive justice, it becomes possible to formulate principles intended to promote distributive justice that should enhance the work of social workers, whatever their practice concentration.[15] For example,

1. The profession and its associated institutions must combat unfair discriminatory practices in the work and attitudes of their constituents or be censured for participating in the perpetration of the disadvantages they entail.

This principle is formulated so as to deny the possibility of a neutral stance toward inequities. It assumes that one cannot enter the stream of community life and remain dry; nor can one avoid some deflection of its flow. The worker either imparts the principle in her practice or departs from it; her

15. Lewis, "Morality and the Politics of Practice."

actions provide the evidence by which her adherence to the principle can be judged.

2. Institutional restrictions that limit opportunities, as well as the personal shortcomings of recipients that may curtail his options, are legitimate targets for change.

This principle carries the implicit expectation that the worker will be knowledgeable both in actions intended to change institutional structures and in actions intended to structure personal and interpersonal change. It does not assume that these actions need be separate or qualitatively distinctive. The principle further recognizes that institutional arrangements in troubled communities must not model professional and organizational goals but serve them. If the profession is to act in accordance with its commitment to distributive justice, it must be prepared to transform both itself and other community institutional structures and agencies employing social workers.

This principle also visualizes the societal and personal components in every service encounter. In seeking to maximize the recipient's utilization of resources, the worker focuses on the personal and social restraints that determine the current opportunities available to the recipient. She would be so directed whatever the nature of the recipient's problems, whatever their etiologies. Utilization of service appears in practice as action; and in the context of the helping process, it is an important form of social action. It is not likely to be enhanced unless the recipient becomes involved on his own behalf. It cannot be enhanced where the opportunities available for improved utilization are so limited that they deny choice.

3. Opportunities to participate in the development of programs, in the formulation of policies and proce-

dures, and in the practice decisions directly affecting their lives must be afforded to the disadvantaged as a minimal expectation of organizations and practices intended to help them.

It makes little sense to treat individuals and institutions as the beneficiaries of a service while denying them a central role in its development. This principle therefore requires organizations and professionals intent upon helping people to include those for whom their services are intended in all phases of the process whereby needs are identified and resources are organized and distributed to meet those needs. The knowledge basis for the propositional element in this principle has received extensive documentation in the literature of social work, particularly as a result of the antipoverty, community mental health, and recipient self-help programs. This principle does not require that those intended to benefit directly from the program have control of it, but it does not exclude this possibility. There is increasing evidence that many recipient groups favor such control, and experience may prove that it is an essential ingredient for sound practice. It is conceivable that recipient control may provide one of the more important opportunities, which traditionally have been denied, to the disadvantaged in our country.

The three principles cited here can be generalized to include a variety of immoral practices known to be prevalent in our society—including denial of fair opportunity to racial and religious minorities, to women, to handicapped persons, to the aged, and to the poor. The propositional elements are derived from facts about social institutions and their function in society, about discrimination and its impact on all groups thereby disadvantaged, and about changes that are required if evident inequities in opportunity are to be eliminated. The ethical commendations are derived from the ethical imperative accepted as essential for the achievement of distributive justice and trust. Together, these propositional and ethical statements justify the principles proposed. The experiences of social workers also justify them—in a way that encourages their acceptance in practice.

PERSONAL AND PROFESSIONAL VALUATIONS

IN HER PROFESSIONAL and nonprofessional experiences, the social worker has the opportunity to observe and evaluate all the unjust and untrustworthy practices of the community in which she lives and works. She stores these perceptions of prevalent social inequalities in memory and refers to them when she seeks to understand events and circumstances new to her experience. Certainly life experiences differ among social workers, and such differences extend to the social contexts and circumstances of their encounters with various forms of discrimination. Some workers have been the victims of unfair behavior; others have practiced such behavior without conscious awareness of its implications. Some have undoubtedly rationalized the injustices they observed, attributing inequities to the influence of fate, faith, or fundamental biological differences. Whereas some workers would find support for the suggested practice principles in their total life experiences, others would view them as contradictory to their nonprofessional (and even certain professional) experience.

Workers who could accept these principles in professional practice but deny their applicability to their own extraprofessional behavior would have to cope with serious inner-directed conflict. One supposes that the mental compartmentalization of behavior norms that must accompany such contradictory directives can be successfully maintained only when it is reinforced by external influences. Social structures, community norms, and institutions generally appear to facilitate and reinforce the mental compartmentalization of behavioral roles by supporting differential role expectations in different settings. Increased dependence on such external structures to sustain mental compartmentalizations would ultimately deprive the worker of considerable freedom to respond imaginatively to recipient need and reinforce a more rigid, habituated, rule-dominated practice. This is a heavy price to pay, but it is probably unavoidable if inner-directed conflict is to be controlled.

Experience teaches us to accept as a matter of fact the ability of most persons to engage in inconsistent behavior; we accept it as normal so long as contradictory behaviors are not simultaneously evident in the same social context. If a helping profession (and its associated institutions) promotes such inconsistencies, however, it cannot expect to compartmentalize them so readily. Policies and procedures in an institution are never entirely private; the tensions generated by contradictory policies are communicated to both the practitioner and the recipients, and they are unlikely to be fully absorbed in intraorganizational stresses and strains. The profession can hardly afford to be inconsistent in its principled behavior lest it be judged dishonest to the point where its rules subvert professed intentions. If inconsistent behavior in professional and personal activities can deplete the energy and resources of an individual, it can have an even more disastrous effect on a profession.

»» ««

Our analysis of intellectual tools, theory, and ethical imperatives inevitably leads us to the ultimate intellectual aids that imbue these tools with their power to affect practice: knowledge and values. Lacking the power that knowledge and values impart to them, actions are meaningless and pointless. In the next two chapters, I consider first knowledge as it affects skill and then values.

»»   ««

CHAPTER SIX

Knowledge

THE WORKER WHO HAS MASTERED the rules and principles of her practice soon discovers that they are necessary but insufficient to guide action in the variety of situations in which her help is sought. When she seeks further enlightenment in theory and ethics, she learns that they too are helpful but do not cover all situations in the guidance they offer. Theory and ethics rely on other sources for their strength as conceptual tools: Theories depend upon the truths they explain; and ethics upon values. At this point, the worker may be pleased to learn that the relation of knowledge and values to her practice has received more attention in professional literature than have rules, principles, theory, and ethics.[1] But

1. For discussions of relevant issues, see R. Clyde White, "The Problem of Knowing in Social Work," *Social Work* 1, no. 4 (October 1956): 94–99; Ernest Greenwood, "Social Science and Social Work: A Theory," *Social Service Review* 29, no. 1 (March 1955): 20–33; Catherine S. Chilman, "Production of New Knowledge of Relevance to Social Work and Social Welfare," *Social Work Education Reporter* 17, no. 3 (September 1969): 49–57; *Building Social Work Knowledge*, Report of a Conference (New York: National Association of Social Workers, 1964); William E. Gordon, "Toward a Social Work Frame of Reference," *Journal of Education for Social Work* 1, no. 2 (Fall 1965): 19–26; idem, "Knowledge and Value: Their Distinction and Relationship in Clarifying Social Work," *Social Work* 10, no. 3 (July 1963): 32–39; Walter L. Kindelsperger, "An Inquiry into the Anatomy of Social Work

she will quickly discover that this attention does not insure that the relationship has been clearly defined.

She will find that despite agreement on the need to employ knowledge from other professions, from the human sciences, and from the humanities, there is no consensus on the criteria for selecting what knowledge might be relevant or on the means of formulating this knowledge for use in her work.[2] Some authorities maintain that social work has shown

Knowledge." mimeographed (New York, Council on Social Work Education, Committee on Advanced Education in Social Work, April 1967); Sheila B. Kamerman, Ralph Dolgoff, George Getzel, and Judith Nelsen, "Knowledge for Practice: Social Science in Social Work," in *Shaping the New Social Work*, ed. Alfred J. Kahn (New York: Columbia University Press, 1973), pp. 97–147; Martin Rein and Sheldon H. White, "Knowledge for Practice," *Social Service Review* 55 (March 1981): 1–41; William J. Reid, "Mapping the Knowledge Base of Social Work," *Social Work* 26, no. 2 (March 1981): 124–32; Joel Fischer, "The Social Work Revolution," *Social Work* 26, no. 3 (May 1981); 199–209.

2. Edwin J. Thomas, "Selecting Knowledge from Behavioral Science," in *Building Social Work Knowledge,* pp. 39–47; Herbert M. Aptekar, "Relevant Knowledge in Advanced Education for Social Work" (Paper presented at Spring Workshop of the Advisory Committee on Advanced Education in Social Work, Council on Social Work Education, Riverdale, N.Y., April 12–15, 1976); Martin Bloom, "The Selection of Knowledge from the Behavioral Sciences and Its Integration into Social Work Curricula," *Journal of Education for Social Work* 5, no. 1 (Spring 1969): 15–27; Catherine S. Chilman, "Production of New Knowledge of Relevance to Social Work and Social Welfare: An Examination of Knowledge Which Underlies Social Work Practice and Permeates the Curriculum," *Social Work Education Reporter* 17, no. 3 (1968): 49–57; John A. Crane, "Utilizing the Fundamentals of Science in Educating for Social Work Practice," *Journal of Education for Social Work* (Fall 1966): 22–29; Alfred Kadushin, "The Knowledge Base of Social Work," in *Issues in American Social Work*, ed. Alfred J. Kahn (New York: Columbia University Press, 1959), pp. 38–79; Herman D. Stein, "Social Science in Social Work Practice and Education," *Social Casework* 36, no. 4 (April 1955): 147–55; *Putting Knowledge to Use: A Distillation of the*

more interest in communicating a body of knowledge supposed to exist than in verifying or advancing this knowledge.[3] Others differ over the merits of empirical knowledge versus personal,[4] of understanding knowledge versus use.[5] For good reason, then, she is likely to turn to her own work experience for some assistance in clarifying what she needs to know.

During a typical work day, the social worker is brought into close contact with persons seeking assistance and expecting action. She is repeatedly involved in establishing, sustaining, or terminating interpersonal relationships. Her immediate experiences loom large, and her perceptions and evaluations—based upon what she has seen, heard, and experienced—can be expected to encourage sense-oriented

Literature Regarding Knowledge Transfer and Change (Los Angeles: Human Interaction Research Institute, in collaboration with National Institute of Mental Health—Mental Health Services Developmental Branch, Rockville, Md., 1976); Martin Bloom, *The Paradox of Helping: Introduction to the Philosophy of Scientific Practice* (New York: John Wiley & Sons, 1975), pp. 89–99; Allen Rubin and Aaron Rosenblatt, eds. *Sourcebook on Research Utilization* (New York: Council on Social Work Education, 1979).

3. Clyde R. White, "The Problems of Knowing in Social Work," *Social Work* 1, no. 4 (October 1956): 94–99; Samuel Finestone, "The Scientific Component in the Casework Field Curriculum," *Social Casework* 36, no. 5 (May 1955): 195–202.

4. Rosa Wessel, "The Meaning of Professional Education for Social Work," *Social Service Review* 35, no.2 (June 1961: 153–60; Paul Tillich, "The Philosophy of Social work," ibid., 36, no. 1 (March 1962): 13–16.

5. Issac L. Hoffman, "Reasearch, Social Work and Scholarship," *Social Service Review* 30, no. 1 (1956): 20–32; David Fanshel, ed., *Future of Social Work Research* (Washington, D. C.: National Association of Social Workers, 1980), pp. 7–10, gives current proposals to narrow the gap between knowledge production and its use; see also Jack Rothman, "Harnessing Research to Enhance Practice: A Research and Development Model," ibid.; pp. 75–90. Frederick W. Seidel, "Making Research Relevant for Practitioners," in *Future of Social Work Research,* ed. Fanshel, pp. 53–65.

formulations. "I feel," rather than "I think," more appropriately expresses what is actually in her mind as she records a day's observations.

In her work, she also confronts the routine, the ordinary, and the expected, all easily ordered within a previously digested conceptualization. The unanticipated, the bizarre, and the unusual nevertheless intrude significantly; and their unexplained and peculiar characteristics often create engrossing, exhausting, but frequently most demanding interludes. It would be surprising not to find that the records of these workers more often contain the expression of experience, "I believe," than the implied claim to certainty, "I know."

It happens that *believe* and *know* are key terms central to any investigation of the general theory of knowledge. Attempts to define them have posed many of the contentious issues in epistemological scholarship.[6] It would hardly suit the purposes of this analysis to ignore their currency in social work communications and expect the reader to realize the meanings these terms are given here. On the other hand, social work has experienced more than its fair share of confusion from the use of words adopted with the intent to clarify meanings. Rather than coin new words in an effort to avoid confusion with old meanings, definitions used here are borrowed from philosophical texts.[7]

A social worker's belief statement can be a nonjudgmental expression of her state of mind or a judgment about some phenomenon. Where it is the latter, the question, "What proof do you have that what you *believe* is true?" can be disconcerting but nevertheless is justified. If the worker's statement is not intended to offer a judgment but to report

6. Bertrand Russell, *Human Knowledge: Its Scope and Limits* (New York: Simon & Schuster, 1948), pp. 3–9, 142–61.

7. I. Scheffler, *Conditions of Knowledge* (Chicago: Scott, Foresman, 1965); Roderick M. Chisholm, Theory of Knowledge (Englewood Cliffs, N.J.: Prentice-Hall, 1966).

her own internal state, a question calling for proof can be mistaken as a deliberate challenge to the correctness of what only she can know. Sometimes a second question, the corollary to the proof question, asks for evidence gathered and analyzed by methods that conform to acceptable standards of credibility. When such a question is asked about a worker's nonjudgmental statement, both participants in the dialogue may terminate their discussion, each having privately confirmed the futility of attempting to reason with a dogmatic adversary.

A nonsemantic element that pertains to this discussion of the confused meanings associated with belief statements has to do with the strongly held convictions that are central to an understanding of practice. For those who are persuaded that insight and intuition appropriately inform belief and provide the most useful additions to that store of personal knowledge which is relevant in social work practice, "I believe" may simultaneously express an internal state and render a judgment about objective phenomena. The issues posed by those holding to these views transcend terminological differences. For a variety of reasons, and from different perspectives, these views are fairly prevalent among professional social workers.

Belief, adequacy of evidence, and truth are viewed as three conditions for knowing, in the sense of *knowing that.*[8] *Belief,* a disposition to act in certain ways under certain circumstances, can be viewed as a 'theoretical' state characterizing the orientation of the person to the world. *Adequacy of evidence,* determined by judging all available evidence at the time the belief is asserted in accordance with standards of credibility, assumes that the person making the assertion has an evidential argument which he understands. *Truth,* a condition, asserts the existence of the state of affairs about which the belief is held.

8. Scheffler, *Conditions of Knowledge.*

Belief statements that assert more than the directly given and are therefore translatable into predictive statements about objective reality must be distinguished from beliefs that involve no judgments and are therefore not subject to error. The former can be tested by confirmation in direct experience — their consequences are explored in scientific explanations.[9]

For the worker most concerned to learn what is known rather than what is felt, focusing on empirically verifiable assertions about objective reality will prove more helpful. This approach does not exclude reports of self-awareness offered as evidence to deny or affirm some judgment about objective realities. Indeed, personal reports of this sort can logically be expected to meet acceptable standards of credibility, and the judgments they offer can be proved erroneous by an examination of their consequences.[10]

'Truths' held to be self-evident are occasionally questioned. Such doubts occur most often in times of drastic and rapid change, when rules of justice and economy, methods of scientific inquiry, esthetic styles, and promised paths to salvation are being discarded. If doubts are sustained, even 'truths' commanding unquestioned adherence may be toppled from their exalted positions. A society survives such challenges to 'truths' because they rarely occur simultaneously in all areas of its civilization. Some self-evident 'truths' hold firm to provide the fulcrum for overturning others.

Thus some 'truths' survive among our cherished beliefs longer than others. Some are found to be more self-evident than others. As defined earlier, truth expresses the belief that objective realities about which judgments are rendered are sustantive, and not simply mind-made. This is the type of

9. C.I. Lewis, *An Analysis of Knowledge and Valuation* (LaSalle, Ill.: Open Court, 1946, reprinted 1962), pp. 1–23.

10. Michael Polanyi, *Personal Knowledge* (Chicago: University of Chicago Press, 1958) provides an in-depth analysis of personal reports as evidence.

truth whose self-evident nature is assumed in this inquiry.

Knowledge, which (according to our definition) is associated with the apprehension of cognitive and emotive experiences, is responsive to time and circumstance. What we have come to know, of all the possible things that could be known, is in part a reflection of our social history. For social work, as for all other areas of human action, this social context has strongly influenced what it claims as knowledge, and our analysis of social work's knowledge structure must account for it.

Social workers assume that the experiences that constitute their practice, although real, more often than not escape their full understanding. In filling the records they prepare with descriptions of these experiences, they assume that they are properly presenting the significant and recognizable aspects of their practice. Novices in the profession readily appreciate how useful such descriptions can be. These descriptions help them to understand the otherwise unfamiliar in their own work.

Were social workers simply systematic observers seeking to describe their experiences, they would focus on methods that promise more reliable descriptions. But social workers are far more concerned with effecting changes in the circumstances engaging their efforts than they are in describing them. They measure their understanding by the consequences of their actions. The very failure of expected effects to follow from the activities intended to bring them about, in practice raises questions about the completeness of what is known.

The work that requires their special competencies generates the wide range of observations that social workers report. Upon examination, these observations suggest that social workers report external perceptions, memories, self-awareness (reflection or inner consciousness), and reasoning—all commonly accredited sources of genuine knowledge.[11] If we accept such reports as dependable evidence, we also accept that

---

11. Chisholm, *Theory of Knowledge,* p. 57.

the potential exists for developing knowledge from social worker observations.

The activities and characteristics of social workers, the settings in which they work, and the circumstances of their profession have also been observed and described in some detail. These reports provide another potential source of evidence that can be useful in enriching the pool of available knowledge.

The thoughts, feelings, and behavior of people—and the development, organization, and operation of their social institutions—are of interest to social workers. What is known about these areas of human experience that will also be judged germane to social work practice will vary depending on time and place. Observations that provide the basis for evidence in the human sciences and in other professions are recognized sources of knowledge for social work.

A lack of sources is obviously not a critical factor in the development of knowledge from social work practice.

Formidable problems are posed in the observation of the complex and varied phenomena of concern to social workers. Because the efforts of social workers are very often occupied in influencing stressful, crises-ridden situations, their choices of what, when, and how to observe are limited in practice by the demands for service. Persons seeking service, as well as organizations employing social workers, set action priorities that condition what a worker can, will, and wants to observe.

Just exactly how to select those observations that are likely to produce the knowledge social workers can appropriately utilize in their work is not clear. The simple availability of social work practices for reliable observation hardly assures their relevance. The least significant event is often the most amenable to systematic, precise, and accurate observation. Both trivial and routine encounters are the most frequently noted, if only to highlight the significant and unusual. Persistence may simply reflect those natural conditions least subject to change through the efforts of social workers.

The inclinations of the observer can also be expected to influence the choice of what to observe. The combination of opportunity, willingness, and ability to observe—which commonly helps to determine the authenticity of reports—also serves to filter experience through a personal screen that may meet the need of the observer but does not necessarily fill that of the profession.[12] Moreover, the social worker actively shapes the content of what she observes, and this further complicates her observations. As an observing participant, she imparts to each observation her personal style as it influences both the events she helps originate and the report she makes.

Any decision about what to observe will necessarily depend on what is available for observation and who can make the observations; but these influences are appropriately manifest only after a more fundamental condition—that the nature of social work be specified—is met. If we do not know what constitutes the universe to be studied, it is unlikely that we will be able to determine the relevance of experiences for the profession or to arrive at a rational basis for selecting that portion to be deliberately subjected to systematic observation.

Social workers have been and continue to be employed for the administration of the community-sponsored services of social agencies in a manner that will assure the opportunity for their maximum utilization by recipients and those likely to become recipients of their services. Assuming that this function is a useful, *but not a complete* frame of reference for social work practice, the answer to the question, "what is to be known?" can be given in a few words: the social worker needs to know all that is essential to the successful performance of this function.

Because what is essential to successful performance is cir-

12. Louis Gottschalk, *Understanding History: A Primer of Historical Method,* 2d ed. (New York: Alfred A. Knopf, 1969).

cumscribed by the function, this observation directs our search to relevant phenomena. Beyond the prescription of parameters, however, this definition of function offers little guidance for selecting criterion measures of success and even less for determining just which practices are likely to lead to the achievement of service goals. In relation to these short-comings, the definition mirrors the state of knowledge in the profession. No firm answer to either of these questions is currently available.[13] In the absence of such knowledge, it is not surprising that efforts to determine the necessary knowns for practice have not depended on measures of consequences but have instead enumerated what is to be known in light of what is to be done.[14]

Social workers are expected to help people in need and to promote the personal and social changes that will assist in this task. Lists of what the worker must know to fulfill these expectations have been developed, and the worker who takes them seriously is never likely to feel adequate to the work she must do.[15] All the social and behavioral sciences, all the human service professions, as well as research methodologies, communications and linguistics, and all the humanities, appear on one or more of these lists. One concludes that this profession embraces the entire human condition to such an extent that even a renaissance person would be reluctant to engage in it.

Obviously there is a need for some guidance about what to select from such a shopping list; and although such guidance has been offered by a number of scholars, no one has success-

13. "Conceptual Frameworks II," *Social Work* 26, no. 1 (January 1981): 6, 85–93.

14. Scott Briar, "Needed: A Simple Definition of Social Work," *Social Work,* 26, no. 1 (January 1981): 83–84.

15. See, for example, Chilman, "Production of New Knowledge."

fully implemented the steps proposed as necessary for such selection.[16] The difficulties involved are formidable.

The range of the knowns in each of these areas is by no means clear, and those most knowledgeable about each subject note that their disciplines are not yet completely firm about either their findings or their methodologies. Moreover, many of the findings do not apply directly to social work. Even if the worker should successfully identify relevant findings, she would then be confronted with the very difficult task of formulating practice principles based on these findings so that they were useful in guiding her work.

One important concern that might not occur to a worker is whether what is purported to be known does in fact meet the condition for establishing a valid claim. Adequate evidence — relying as it must on methods of derivation, the scope of observations, and the logical connection between the explanation offered and the findings obtained — would have to be demonstrated. Unfortunately, neither the scientist she consults nor an authoritative social work source is likely to provide enlightenment on this score. The worker may end her search for the evidential justification of explanations by concluding in this area, as in many others of her life, faith is a necessary substitute for fact. She will decide to believe that what is asserted is in fact known. As a result of this experience, she may be encouraged to accept as true that which she in reality does not know to be true. She may finally fall back on a dogmatic faith in the givens rather than pursuing the spirit of inquiry that supposedly characterizes the disciplines that developed them.[17]

16. See Edwin J. Thomas, "Beyond Knowledge Utilization in Generating Human Service Technology," in *Future of Social Work Research*, ed. Fanshel, pp. 91–103, for a proposed approach that the author believes offers promise in overcoming these difficulties.

17. Aptekar, "Relevant Knowledge," p. 22.

The worker is likely to assume that mastery of what is supposedly known in the human sciences is primarily a retrieval problem, complicated by a need to translate what is known into useful principles to guide her practice. In her search for some basis upon which to determine the credibility of the claims to knowledge associated with the substantive findings and explanations retrieved, she will find that most social work authorities have accepted them on faith; and she may decide to be equally trusting. Her natural inclination will probably lead her to get on with her work, find out what problem conditions she will have to help change, and determine for herself which of the knowns she happens to locate in her review of such materials are helpful in their solution. Should she follow this inclination, she will have hit upon the most prevalent tactic thus far devised for dealing with these difficulties.

This tactic actually defines the given to be changed as the initial stimulus in the quest for relevant knowledge. Ignoring discipline boundaries, it directs the worker to tap whatever sources are likely to help her deal with a problem. When she confronts the recipient whose problem initiated the search for the known, however, she quickly realizes that the riches retrieved only complicate her primary task—to bring all she knows to bear in this unique situation in a manner that is most relevant to this problem's peculiar attributes.[18]

The other appeal of this tactical approach to knowledge retrieval is methodological. If one ignores the arts of scientific investigation and serendipity, the bulk of scientific work is logically analyzable into distinctive, sequential activities, frequently described as problem solving.[19] The problem-solving approach, in addition to its utility as a framework for

18. Martin Wolins, "Selection of Foster Parents: Early Stages in the Develoment of a Screen" (D.S.W. diss., Columbia University, 1959).

19. William I.B. Beveridge, *The Art of Scientific Investigation* (New York: Random House, 1957).

knowledge retrieval, also suggests a model of procedure to be followed in dealing with the client's problem itself, modeling the form in which help is given to the procedures whereby the knowledge that informs the helper is derived.[20]

It is best to pause at this point to consider the implications of this discussion for the worker. Thus far she has learned that there is a wealth of substantive findings and concepts in the human sciences and humanities for use in her practice and that she wants to master these materials. She has discovered that her task will be essentially one of retrieval and translation. She has learned that a problem-solving approach will provide her with an entry tool to be used in locating what is relevant. She has concluded that she is expected to treat the findings retrieved as knowns though they may appear to her as givens to be accepted on faith. Although she is merely an interpreter of such material, when she seeks to use what she has learned in the practice situation, she must be far more creative.[21] Using her ingenuity and imagination to find effective applications, she may in fact contribute to the development of principles that order such basic knowledge for practice. Finally, she will be encouraged to appreciate the elements of the problem-solving method and to test them out as tools in helping recipients solve their problems. The worker will not fail to appreciate the usefulness of knowledge taken from the human sciences, the humanities, and other professions in orienting her in her practice. Such knowledge locates her practice in time and place and provides her with

20. For an early version of this currently popular approach, see Louis J. Lehrman, "The Scientific Nature of the Social Caseworker's Professional Process," in *Social Work Practice in the Field of Tuberculosis,* ed. Eleanor Cockerill (Pittsburgh: University of Pittsburgh School of Social Work, 1954), pp. 152–62; Eleanor Cockerill, "Implications of the Scientific Method for Medical Social Work," ibid., pp. 163–66.

21. Aptekar, "Relevant Knowledge," p. 22.

guidance in knowing where to look and what to look for. But the worker will still find such knowledge to be of little use in providing her with "how-to" prescriptions — with principles and rules for practice.

In seeking justification for practice principles, she is directed to the theory and ethics that inform them. In seeking justification for the theory, she is directed to the knowledge the theory seeks to explain. Yet when she attempts to reverse the process and tries to derive practice principles from the orienting knowledge base, she is confronted with the resistance of such knowledge to manipulations that try to shape it to the requirements of practice principles. What this confrontation helps her realize (and what is otherwise hidden from her awareness) is that the generalizations of these theoretical sciences differ in fundamental ways from the generalizations of a practice science. Resolving these differences is not only a difficult task; in time, it may also prove to be impossible. The practice science from which the worker will be obliged to draw in order to provide the service her work is intended to deliver will have to inform her how she is to go about doing such work-related tasks as these:

1. Making decisions affecting action in uncertain situations.
2. Engaging in problem solving.
3. Utilizing the case method to define a situation and formulate a plan of action with intention to influence.
4. Basing moral behavior on ethical imperatives derived from a set of relevant values.
5. Appreciating differences and understanding the importance of individualizing situations and persons.
6. Disciplining the idiosyncratic in style.
7. Communicating in a manner that enhances understanding and furthers intentions.
8. Engaging in ongoing self-appraisal.

What is expected in the performance of each of these tasks is detailed in Table 1. The worker soon discovers, however, that although these intellectual skills are necessary, they are hardly sufficient to accomplish the work she is expected to do. She also needs knowledge that orients her to the substantive content of her work. She finds she must be able to do the following:

1. Identify needs and appropriate resources in the area of practice concern.
2. Appreciate the ethical and theoretical foundations that inform the program of services she offers and influence her choice of objectives and methods of work.
3. Recognize the functional relevance of administrative, supervisory, and service-delivery structures and roles in organizational networks that seek to implement progams.
4. Understand the processes whereby the results of practice efforts are accounted for and how additions to practice theory are incorporated into the scope of practice competence.

No worker would want to be ignorant of the substantive content implicit in these tasks; but this knowledge, while necessary, is also insufficient to permit her to engage in a practice.

In any situation where the worker is expected to provide a service, the complicating factor that gives the 'how' its distinctive attributes is the frequency of decisions that require the concurrent coordination of multiple judgments in uncertain and particular situations. The worker is called upon to know how to do the following:

1. Evaluate the relationship of need to resource and arrive at useful definitions of the imbalance to be altered.
2. Design a unit of service whose objectives are realistic and whose implementation is feasible.

3. Implement the program through appropriate administrative, supervisory, and direct practice activities judged likely to achieve program goals and objectives.
4. Develop monitoring procedures that permit an accounting of the effort expended and the purposes accomplished while assisting in systematic evaluations of results.

In relation to each task, there is a critical need to think about the 'how' of practice. As noted earlier, the help that rules and principles provide in how to think about the doing ultimately informs the worker as to what she needs most in her work. Thus the worker will be led to conclude that the core body of knowledge that uniquely prepares her for her particular practice is the sum of these principles and rules.

PERSONAL KNOWLEDGE

IN ADDITION TO that knowledge whose nature permits the form or organization exemplified by rules, principles, and theories, there is also self-awareness — upon which every practicing social worker depends for sensitivity and style in practice. Self-awareness, which is a form of personal knowledge, is composed both of belief statements and of evaluative statements that can be confirmed by the evidence of their consequences.[22] Personal knowledge lends a recognizable shape to practice and provides one of its attractions. Such knowledge infuses the worker's activities with empathy, the source of humane qualities present in the helping relationship.

When the worker reports what she feels, we acquire facts about the worker that can help us understand her. Differences in such reported feelings, for example, help us

22. Polanyi, *Personal Knowledge*, p. 55.

KNOWLEDGE

Table 1. Tasks Involved in Professional Practice

1. Making decisions affecting action in uncertain situations.

   a. Being aware of the structure of explanations in both science and the creative arts to the extent that these enhance or restrict what can be anticipated as realistic alternatives.

   b. Knowing the role of values in conditioning choices in uncertain situations.

   c. Knowing how to develop adequate descriptions of situations that will constitute the context in which decisions are to be made.

   d. Being able to identify, describe, order, and generate alternatives.

   e. Understanding the probabilities and risks entailed in choices of alternatives.

   f. Understanding the conditional nature of both action and the self-correcting process in making a series of decisions over time.

2. Engaging in problem-solving.

   a. Being able to formulate problems in operational terms.

   b. Knowing techniques involved in identifying the dimensions of the problem; in designing an approach to be followed in dealing with the problem; in implementing the design and in reporting the results.

   c. Knowing how to consider alternative approaches to problems.

   d. Understanding how to draw valid and relevant conclusions based on findings of the study process, with special emphasis on the feedback of such conclusions to aid in further problem solving.

   e. Appreciating the ethical considerations involved in the problem-solving process.

3. Utilizing the case method to define a situation and formulate a plan of action with intention to influence.

   a. Developing a life-history of the unit of attention.

   b. Knowing the circumstances that influence the definition of a situation.

   c. Knowing the strengths and limits of the case method in formulating generalizations.

   d. Being able to appropriately modify requirements for case formulations in light of peculiar attributes of the particular situation.

   e. Being able to attribute meaning to continuities and discontinuities in each case.

   f. Being aware of the influence of both self and method on the reliability and validity of inferences based on a case.

4. Basing moral behavior on ethical imperatives derived from relevant values.

   a. Understanding the structure of values as they enter practice to influence action.

   b. Knowing the policy implications of ultimate value preferences, including their role in selecting outcome success measures.

   c. Being able to identify commendations that derive from ethical imperatives and to understand how they influence principled practice.

   d. Knowing the nature, structure, and role of ethical codes and appreciating their effects on standards of, from, and for practice.

   e. Being aware of the societal and personal value preferences that affect choices.

5. Appreciating differences and understanding the importance of individualizing situations and persons.

    a. Requiring a sense of history — both societal and personal — to appreciate how cultures, institutions, and people are shaped by their peculiar experiences.

    b. Understanding innovation and creativity to appreciate the influence of personal and social effort in shaping both.

    c. Knowing the physical, interpersonal, and societal constraints that differentially advantage and disadvantage cultures and people.

    d. Skillfully ascertaining the significance of unique features in otherwise common events that define what makes them different. Similarly, achieving this understanding with persons and institutions.

    e. Developing self-awareness to appreciate and control for one's own differences when intervening in the lives and circumstances of others, so as not to burden them with what is not helpful in such differences.

6. Disciplining the idiosyncratic in style.

    a. Understanding what is entailed in completing what one sets out to do — neither going beyond it nor falling short of it. Limiting oneself to what is worth expressing through action. Eliminating the insignificant to focus on what is fundamental — the process of simplification.

    b. Knowing how to organize in a definite manner parts or elements into a larger unit — a whole.

    c. Knowing the limits of what is to be worked with.

    d. Knowing one's limits and how to employ these to enhance one's unique use of means and methods, freeing oneself to do what comes easily and naturally.

    e. Placing oneself in the background — attending to the substance of the service, the mood and temper of the person served rather than those of the provider of service.

    f. Becoming willing to see criticism and failure not as signs of weakness or defeat but as very probable outcomes when actions must be taken in uncertain situations; viewing them both as potential sources for reducing their occurrence in future efforts.

7. Communicating in a manner that enhances understanding.

  a. Using language (both verbal and nonverbal) skillfully.

  b. Knowing media, their strengths and limitations; being able to employ them when appropriate.

  c. Understanding the range of audiences to be reached and their preferred modes of communication.

  d. Being able to speak and write clearly and to employ appropriate imagery to convey meanings in a simple and direct fashion.

  e. Knowing the networks through which communications are channeled, and the noise, feedback, and modulations that accompany their use; how transmission can be simplified and reception enhanced.

  f. Appreciating the power of information, the ethical issues involved in its control, and the limits on the acceptable uses of such control in a moral practice.

8. Engaging in ongoing self-appraisal.

  a. Origins: Knowing one's own cultural and social history.

  b. Style: Appreciating one's preference in ways of learning, work, and play.

  c. Status: Perceiving one's location in community, group, and interpersonal hierarchical arrangements.

  d. Stance: Determining one's involvement with and response to authority, ideologies, individual and group differences.

  e. Sensitivities: Understanding one's moods, tempos, tastes, as these affect service-related relationships.

distinguish among workers in many decisive respects. For example, workers who report emotional trauma when brought into close and persistent contact with severely handicapped persons are unlikely to be assigned to work with paraplegics. Nor do we ignore similar traumatic reactions to environmental stimuli in offering guidance and support to the worker in the use of self in practice. Obviously, we do not approach such statements merely to note their prevalence. We use them to appreciate each person's capacity to experience the emotions she reports. Concerned as we must be with the practice implications of these feelings, we necessarily place them in a framework that suggests their possible consequences for the recipients of service. In this respect, from the perspective of professional usage such facts are incorporated into evaluative belief statements so they can be verified by the evidence of their consequences.

For an individual experiencing such feelings, they have added meaning. They constitute her emotional life. They are manifest in the pain, the sorrow, the joy, the pleasure she knows personally; they represent a part of her existence whose impact is present a priori in the life that follows. Like all others who bother to consider such matters, workers know that their feelings influence their choices, affect their decisions, and demand to be taken into account in their practice. Workers who are not aware of the manner in which the consequences of these feelings are evidenced in practice can be helped to an awareness of their influence. A worker may know she reacts negatively to hostility in a recipient, and she may consciously try to manage her behavior to compensate for the undesirable effects of her reactions in practice. She may not realize, however, that her overall caseload shows a fairly consistent pattern of missed appointments with hostile recipients but no such pattern with recipients who reach out to her for her support. In this instance, the worker can evaluate her feelings to make a judgment about their consequences for her own practice, and this judgment is subject to confirmation based on observable evidence. It is as necessary to account for such personal knowledge as it is to account for other forms of knowledge in any scheme purporting to describe how knowledge influences practice. Failure to do so would limit our understanding of what must be known in order to explain practice.

Personal knowledge is also of concern in a theory of practice. The comment that "in the last analysis, the practitioner of an art must discover the heart of the whole matter for himself," suggests that synthesis may be more valuable than analysis in a worker's attempt to understand the personal dimensions of practice.[23] This analysis recognizes the importance of personal and private awareness in practice but suggests that these become knowable as fact whenever they enter to affect the helping relationship. Although we need not relegate the art of practice to a realm beyond knowing explanations, we may remain unknowing about the manner in which the esthetic originates in the person.

>» «<

Without enumerating all one may want to know in order to do, but recognizing the essential intellectual skills and core uses to which knowledge and such skills will be put, I have tried to describe how the worker assimilates beliefs and 'know-that' statements into her practice. I have also recognized the importance of personal knowledge for the worker. Chapter 7 considers the peculiar attributes of values as they affect the worker and her practice.

23. Mary Richmond, *Social Diagnosis* (New York: Russel Sage Foundation, 1917), p. 103.

»» ««

CHAPTER SEVEN

Values

CHOICES ARE INEVITABLE in the exercise of professional judgment, and practice decisions make such judgments unavoidable. Informed judgments are preferable to those based on ignorance, and purposeful judgments to those not directed to a desired goal. We have considered the manner in which the directives in rules, the propositions in principles, and theories seek to organize, husband, and facilitate the communication of knowledge for use in practice. We have similarly analysed the manner in which the commands in rules, the commendations in principles, and ethics seek to organize, husband, and facilitate the communication of values. We must now complete the latter with a discussion of values, from which ultimate purposes are derived.

VALUE JUDGMENTS

BELIEF, as a form of knowing, has served as an aspect of explanation that is devoid of ethical conviction. We were thus intentionally able to consider how the worker must arrive at truthful descriptions and explanations, not how they might be favored or disfavored.[1] This latter interest is addressed in

---

1. Charles L. Stevenson, *Ethics and Language,* (New Haven: Yale University Press, 1944), p. 4.

Chapter 5, where imperatives, commendations, and commands are considered. Because ethical imperatives are justified by reference to values, they pose additional issues that a worker must confront in her practice.

Value terms are complex. They incorporate criteria and standards by which the value conveyed is to be recognized in concrete instances. They also relate such specifics to the generic class of commendations to which the term is applicable.[2] The standards entailed in a value term that is used to judge a situation in which choice is possible serve to inform in a manner not unlike the information-giving function performed by statements of fact. It is in their evaluative function that value terms evidence preferences not found in truth statements. This commendation attribute of value terms provides the basis for a definition of value judgment that will be assumed in this discussion. We will assume that when a social worker in her practice decides she ought to do X and that she recognizes that if she assents to this judgment, she must also assent to the command "Let me do X," then she is exercising a value judgment.[3]

To act, to engage in some sensible action, is to attempt the realization of something worthwhile or the avoidance of something undesirable. This expectation of a result is the intent of the act and the intent of the social worker in adopting it.[4] The *something* to which positive value is ascribed in social work may be the worth, dignity, and welfare of individuals and their responsibility for contributing to the common good.[5] Such values are knowable a priori by analysis of

2. R.M. Hare, *The Language of Morals* (Oxford: At the Clarendon Press, 1952), p. 133.

3. Ibid., pp. 168–69.

4. C.I. Lewis, *An Analysis of Knowledge and Valuation* (La Salle, Ill: Open Court, 1946, reprinted 1962), p. 366.

5. Werner W. Boehm, "The Nature of Social Work," in *Perspectives*

their meaning as it is formulated in definitions. It is possible that such definitions can be either incorrect in their designations or inappropriately applied, but they are not readily subject to empirical confirmation. Without criteria by which the presence or absence of these values can be recognized in specific instances, however, there is little possibility of establishing their presence in the structure of the product that results from practice decisions. These values may in fact be subscribed to without ever appearing in the normative behavior of the worker. In social work practice, it is precisely this possibility that one wishes to avoid.

It is regrettable that the norms evidenced in the work performed by social workers often deviate from supposedly shared professional values. In practice, choices are often made because restricted resources require that the worker do what she knows she can do rather than what she would prefer to do. When a worker is advised that as a member of the profession she ought to assist the recipients of service into independence and help them to realize their fullest potential, she often doubts that the actual service she is free to offer is capable of achieving this end. She can work to overcome stresses that hinder such a realization and try to develop social conditions that encourage the fullest life possible, but she must wonder whether such universal advice is more myth than reality. Although she may believe that in advancing the welfare of recipients she is serving the general welfare of society, she may find herself compelled to engage in activities whose consequences appear inconsistent with this belief.

The statement, "Each person has the right to self-fulfillment, deriving from his inherent capacity and thrust toward that goal,"[6] remains devoid of significance for choices

---

on Social Welfare, ed. Paul E. Weinberger (Toronto: The Macmillan Co., 1969), p. 267.

6. Ibid.

requiring value judgments in practice, unless it can be so formulated as to suggest criteria by which its application can be recognized and its consequences verified. Should such a formulation prove possible, the assessments based on this value preference are knowable in all those respects that any fact may become known. The value *self-fulfillment* becomes significant for choices involving value judgments in practice when it is specified through some criteria such as the following: maintaining one's health, achieving success at work, participating in recreational activities, and the like. These criteria, never exhaustive and always subject to change, may be evidenced in experiencing no loss of time from school or work because of hospitalization or confining illness at home; continued employment because of adequate performance, or promotion on the job because of unusual achievement; or active participation in sports. In these circumstances, her total statement confronts the practitioner with the uncertainties characteristic of professional choices. For example, it may become necessary to institutionalize a person whose condition requires special care. In so doing, the social worker weighs the importance of supplementing depleted abilities against the restrictions in self-fulfillment that institutionalization will entail and chooses on the basis of the anticipated results. It may be true that all choices in practice involve such contingent value judgments. Should this prove to be the case, understanding what contingent situations imply for practice becomes essential to any theory intended to justify it. Whether clear or ambiguous, however, choices can be considered informed only when the worker's predictions about consequences are valid.

It is nevertheless generally true that in seeking directives about what to do it is best to stay with facts. Although in social work—where the effects of action often remain unknown—choices based upon fact could readily exclude reference to rules of conduct, this appears rarely to be the case. In practice, a social worker presumes that there are certain differences in the effects that follow a particular choice among alternatives; and in this sense, she subscribes to the imperative dictated by those presumed effects. One can reasonably assume that she would prefer effects that further her goals over those that do not, and this assumption can be empirically validated. The worker's choice in practice situations thus involves judgments—decisions of principle—even when the worker does not know, but only believes, that certain consequences may follow.[7]

Although the social worker whose values correspond to those accepted by the agency, by the profession, and by her own feelings is likely to have fewer problems in making such judgments, exact correspondence is unlikely in practice. Our society rewards the advantaged at some cost to the disadvantaged; and as a consequence, even in the human service professions, the better able and socially privileged tend to receive higher quality services. In its code of ethics, the social work profession gives the recipient's interests highest priority in making decisions and opposes on principle preferences that work to the disadvantage of the less able and the socially deprived.[8] In this respect, the profession appears to assume that unequal benefits in the provision of social services can be justified only if they contribute to a scheme that improves the expectations of those least advantaged among potentially eligible recipients.[9] When an agency sanctioned by the community does not act in accordance with such a scheme because community practice rewards the able and socially advantaged without improving the expectations of the least advantaged,

7. Hare, *Language of Morals*, p. 70.

8. Harold Lewis, "The Client's Interest," mimeographed (New York: Hunter College School of Social Work, 1980).

9. Donald S. Howard, *Social Welfare: Values, Means, and Ends* (New York: Random House, 1969), p. 391.

that agency may in fact be insisting on choices that run counter to the professional ethic.[10] It does so, for example, when it restricts intake to certain groups; limits direct relief allocations; circumscribes the use of staff time and effort; curtails the scope of problems to be confronted; or introduces other requirements made necessary by limited resources. In practice, such policies often lead to decisions that discriminate in favor of the more advantaged; and as available resources are consumed for the benefit of the best situated, the expectations of the disavantaged are probably reduced in like amount. In such circumstances, an agency's practice can not easily be reconciled with professional ethics.

But even in situations where both the profession and the agency agree on principles, the social worker may disagree with both on the basis of her own personal preferences. For example, she may believe that birth-control techniques should not be shared with recipients because their use is sacrilegious although both her profession and her agency maintain that offering this choice to recipients encourages a form of behavior that can only enhance each recipient's opportunities to realize his or her capacity for self-fulfillment. Such differences are not easily reconciled.

Because it is possible to study the consequences of the actions associated with alternatives, it should be possible to distinguish empirically between those value judgments that have a greater probability of achieving the purposes of programs and those that are self-defeating. Once they achieve the status of fact, such judgments cease to entail imperatives and become givens—assumptions accepted as sociological or psychological truth. At one time, social workers were commended to include a recipient in making decisions that

10. Richard W. Scott, "Professional Employees in a Bureaucratic Structure: Social Work," in *The Semi-Professions and Their Organization,* ed. Amitai Etzioni (New York: Free Press, 1969), p. 131.

affected him on the grounds that such a practice is consistent with a recipient's right of self-determination. This practice has gradually come to be justified on the basis of evidence that the recipient is more likely to implement such decisions if he is included in making them. If the latter understanding achieves the status of fact, the need to include the recipient in the arriving at decisions that affect him will be treated as a given and acted on accordingly. By assessing the consequences of value judgments, we change such judgments from imperatives to facts and contribute to a continuing dynamic between judgments and practice.

STRUCTURE

VALUES PASS FROM ONE distinctive ordered level to another as they are transformed from designations of belief to practice guides in professional activities. These levels have been labeled in terms of the requirement they place on the worker who seeks to implement their intentions. The level furthest from action comprises the set of values that designates a moral perspective. One step closer to action are the ethical imperatives, which—as we have noted—formulate the behavioral requirements through which value sets may be realized. Still closer to action are the commendations incorporated in principles of practice, which specify the manner in which imperatives are to be applied in practice. Finally, closest to action are commands, which are codified into rules and gain their authority as directives from the principles they are intended to realize.

The context of practice helps to shape behavioral norms. Personal, professional, and agency beliefs shape value designations. Contexts of belief and practice thus influence the substance and form of designations and actions. It is apparent that commands go unheeded when their consequences contradict purpose. If it is justified on the basis of normative requirements in performance, such a failure to observe the rules transmits the need for changes at the commendation and imperative levels. In this respect, the feedback from practice to values closely resembles the pattern described earlier for knowledge.

Within any one level, the election of requirements to be met varies from person to person, from agency to agency, and from one area of professional practice to another, so long as contradictory prescriptions are avoided and justification in relation to the dominant value is maintained. Each level organizes its statements independent of the other levels, and each must be understood in terms of its particular mode of expression.[11]

COMMANDS

IN THE EARLIER DISCUSSION OF RULES, I noted that in their application rules do not necessarily operationalize the values and knowledge that justify an agency's program. This can happen, for example, when a social worker implements their formal requirements but misses the spirit of their intent. From the wording of a rule, one can determine neither what guiding principle justifies its application in a particular instance, nor what values commend it as an imperative, nor what propositional assumptions inform it. Such a restriction in wording is understandable, since rules (taken separately) are commands and directives to be followed, not propositions to be justified. From a set of rules, however, it is possible to deduce an intended consequence of their sequential or concurrent application upon the product sought. Thus, in the

11. Mario Bunge, "Metaphysics, Epistemology and Methodology of Levels," in *Hierarchical Structures,* ed. Lancelot Law Whyte, Albert C. Wilson, and Conna Wilson (New York: American Elsevier, 1969), p. 289.

example of rules cited in Chapter 3, rules 2 and 3 both seek to assure that the parents of neglected children have the opportunity to be informed about the expectations of the agency and share with the agency their own expectations. If additional rules provide similar assurances, one can infer from them an underlying principle: Help should be given in such a way as to assure opportunities for both the worker and the recipient to know their mutual expectations, insofar as these are judged likely to affect the outcome of service. Commending as it does a sharing of expectations, this principle discourages the behaviors and attitudes that hinder such sharing simply because they are contrary to the spirit of the commendation. It is necessary for a set of rules to impart to a worker some such implicit guiding principle if a principled practice is to result. It is also necessary for the worker in each instance of task performance to be aware of the foundation of value and knowledge upon which the principle rests. Without this awareness, the worker may apply the rule in a manner that denies its moral justification.

A set of rules presented in an agency manual is generally accompanied by a preamble intended to clarify the reasons and beliefs justifying the rules that follow and the purposes they are expected to achieve. Reliance on written preambles alone, however, is risky in a professional practice, where confusion may be increased by the complexity of the situations in which rules are applied. For this reason, case examples and programmed exposure to selected experiences under skilled supervision are frequently used to illustrate both a sensible and sensitive application of the rule in sound practice and the attributes associated with mistaken applications. By experiencing a critical evaluation of rule application, the worker learns to internalize its meaning in relation to her own peculiar style, so that implementing it becomes natural to her way of work.

I noted earlier that rules can be applied inappropriately (or not at all in processes that are faulted by such omissions) or as a habitual response to situations no longer calling for their use. To guard against such pitfalls, agencies expend considerable time and thought in formulating rules, subjecting them to critical appraisal in the light of the consequences of their application, and assuring their timely revision as conditions of practice change. When agencies routinely recognize these sources of deviant practice, they are likely to modify their practice on the basis of principles whenever minor heresies occur rather than permitting disruptions in practice. Major challenges to the rules are then more readily recognized for what they truly intend, changes in agency programs and practice that stem from the introduction of new principles and require a radically different set of rules.

The command not obeyed fails of its purpose. A command half-heartedly obeyed is evidently less than convincing. No command is less likely to be obeyed than one that fails to achieve its desired results. Many factors can contribute to such failures, including inadequate resources, limited talent, untoward circumstance; but commands are supposedly formulated in the anticipation of such factors and expected to safeguard practice from such unfortunate influences.

In a conflict between rule and result, result will prevail. The rule will be shoved aside by the corrective pressure of unrealized intentions. Initially, pressure will be directed toward the behavior prescribed by the rule: Attempts will be made to modify, add, or drop the tasks it requires in order to overcome its deficiencies. When these changes fail to improve the results of practice, either the propositions or the commendations or both elements of the practice principle justifying the rule will be challenged. We have already considered how such challenges affect propositions. Let us now consider how doubts about commendations may similarly alter practice principles.

Moral judgments that express individual beliefs are matters of fact that pertain to the individuals whose opinions are expressed. As such, they make no predictions; and they are not subject to empirical verification on the basis of their consequences. When such judgments are intended as predictions, they assume the attributes of 'beliefs' whose status as fact can be determined by procedures that meet acceptable standards for establishing truths. Challenges to rules or commands that originate with failures to achieve practice goals are assumed by their advocates to be 'truths' confirmed by experiential evidence. Such challenges cast doubt upon the causal assumptions associated with the commendation that justified the command. One can deal with such challenges at the rule level so long as rule-modification and rule-exception also incorporate additional commands appropriate to the lessons gleaned from disappointing results. Commands that increasingly depend on such modifications, however, begin to lose their authority; and in time they must appeal to higher authority to retain whatever control they seek to impose. For this reason, where commendations and propositions blend theory and ethics into professional guidelines, at the level of practice principles, the critical struggle between behavioral norms (means) and professed ethical imperatives (ends) will be joined.[12]

COMMENDATIONS AND IMPERATIVES

DIRECTIVES TO ACT in certain ways receive their empirical justification from tested hypotheses, that both predict and are confirmed in their predictions. At the level of principle, however, commendations to act in certain ways are further justified by ethical imperatives that suggest the models of

12. Nina Toren, "Semi-Professionalism and Social Work: A Theoretical Perspective," in *The Semi-Professions,* ed. Etzioni, p. 184.

behavior for which these commendations provide action guidelines. Imperatives thus serve to harden attachments to commendations in a manner that is not characteristic of attachments to explanatory propositions. The model of the ethical social work practice conveyed by imperatives prescribes what is to be judged good and what characterizes good practice. Imperative statements of this type are intended to formulate ends beyond those that can be confirmed by the consequences of practice. At the level of principle, they join commendations with an adhesive stronger than the parts they join. Such imperatives indeed have the holding power of faith. For this reason, a challenge to a commendation threatens more than the rules it may alter or the program it may overturn. Such a challenge casts doubts upon the beliefs that have justified fields of service.

It thus may appear far less divisive to a profession to discard propositions than to overturn commendations. Such changes typically affect methods and problem formulations rather than purpose. The scientific ethic assumes that knowledge is both tentative and partial; and the rules for the rejection of knowledge claims are fairly well established. When propositions are dropped because they have been proven false, a scientific imperative is served. One of the intended outcomes of empirical research is indeed that of disproving propositions.

The rules for rejecting commendations, which are justified by imperatives taken as matters of faith, are not so well established. A rejected commendation threatens the ethic itself. It is therefore to be expected that commendations will change more slowly than propositions, ethical imperatives more slowly than theories, and values far more slowly than knowledge. Although it is not uncommon for different (and sometimes contradictory) theories to be used simultaneously to justify both propositions and the methods they prescribe, it is far less probable that different codes of ethics (particularly contradictory ones) will be simultaneously used to justify similar commendations and commands. In general, a profession can tolerate far more challenges to its means than to its ends. Nevertheless, because means and ends are joined in statements of principles in the social work profession, changes in the one cannot easily be insulated from changes in the other.

NORMS

AT THE LEVEL of value designations, where ideology is formulated, justification for ethical imperatives can be found. A consideration of such imperatives thus requires an examination of the way in which the values that justify professional goals are themselves influenced by prevailing norms.

In any society, a fundamental claim for resources to provide the sustenance needed to assure the survival of its population takes precedence over all others. We know that although a society can survive without providing sustenance for all its members, decisions about who shall survive when scarcity prevails (except perhaps in periods of catastrophe and holocaust) are rarely left to the whim of individuals.[13] The prevailing system of allocation is in fact expected to serve as a self-regulating mechanism and insure against societal self-annihilation.[14] Thus that part of the population likely to remain at risk because of inadequate food, clothing, or shelter is determined only in part by the resources available. As a society achieves relative affluence and develops the capacity to meet the needs of persons previously denied allocations,

13. James F. Childress, "Who Shall Live When Not All Can Live?" in *Ethics and Health Policy*, ed. Robert M. Veatch and Roy Bruson (Cambridge, Mass.: Ballinger, 1976), pp. 199–209.

14. Gene Outka, "Social Justice and Equal Access to Health Care," in *Ethics and Health Policy*, ed. Veatch and Bruson, pp. 79–97.

minimal sustenance for increasing numbers of persons may be provided, so long as the distribution mechanism is designed to capitalize on this achievement.

In the United States, for example, grinding poverty and severe deprivation remain matters of both fact and concern, despite the frequent assertion that the nation is now capable of eliminating such deficiencies. If it is true that there are in fact adequate resources, we must therefore conclude that continued widespread deprivation shows that the system of allocation is at fault. It may be that prevailing principles of distribution, developed as they were to cope with the conditions of scarcity, are inappropriate to a society whose resources have become abundant. Titmus appears to appreciate the implications of this possibility when he observes that "Science and technology in alliance with other structuraland demographic changes underway in our societies will callfor a major shift in values; for new incentives and new forms of reward unrelated to the productivity principles, for new criteria applied to the distribution of resources which are not tied to individual 'success' as a measure; for new forms of socially approved 'dependencies'."[15]

It may be inevitable that changing societal conditions will generate beliefs that challenge the 'truths' on which prevailing values depend for their justification. The failure of a society to live up to its potential for human good understandably raises doubts about the principles of distribution on which it relies.

Most reasoning people want justice, security, knowledge, beauty, and self-respect for themselves; and they normally want the same for others if their own opportunities for realiz-

---

15. Richard Titmuss, "Social Welfare and the Art of Giving," in *Socialist Humanism: An International Symposium,* ed. Erich Fromm (New York: Doubleday, Anchor Books, 1966), p. 391.

ing them are thereby enhanced.[16] The quest for these expectations provides the political, economic, scientific, esthetic, and religious realms of a society with the basic motivations justifying human effort. People appear to make decisions concerning work to be done and allocations to be made under ordinary circumstances on the basis in some measure of the interaction of the norms governing choices in each of these realms. A sensible mechanism of distribution would operate in a manner calculated to maximize human good for all and take advantage of the motivations provided by what people want.

In the United States, for the majority of persons seeking the aid of social service agencies and for others whose wants are in certain respects unfulfilled, this mechanism appears to be inoperative. The popular belief that "beggars can't be choosers" reflects the truth of this assertion. Social and economic inequalities create further disadvantages for the dependent; prevailing social and cultural barriers also prejudice opportunities; and discrimination on the basis of race, sex, and age denies equal access to a wide range of positions and offices. Our country's norms for allocating its resources thus appear to fall short of those ethical imperatives that might assure social justice.

A cardinal assumption of our welfare structure — and of the social service programs it promotes — is the belief that the social resources devoted to these programs will help compensate for such injustices in distribution through efforts toward redistribution. The ideologies of welfare in the United States proclaim liberty and opportunity, income and health, education and esthetic satisfaction, and self-respect for all persons

---

16. Paul Schrecker, *Work and History: An Essay on the Structure of Civilization* (New York: Crowell, 1971), develops this theme as a basic assumption for an analysis of civilization.

as their goals. Working within the welfare structure, social work professes similar intentions and justifies them on the basis of values that commit each worker to the worth, dignity, and welfare of each individual and to his responsibility for contributing to the common good. If the imperatives set forth in the profession's code of ethics were completely followed, they could contribute to righting the wrongs imposed by an unjust distributive system and preventing the perpetration of injustice in the welfare enterprise itself. In its claimed values and goals, the profession thus seeks to correct injustice; it asks both itself and the society that sanctions its efforts to provide a principled, just way of distributing human goods.

Professional ethics notwithstanding, the social service agencies that employ social workers are keenly sensitive to the imperatives underlying the distributive mechanisms of the wider community. This attitude is inevitable—community norms are reflected in the budgets approved for programs, and agency policies are responsive to budget limitations. The social worker whose efforts on behalf of the recipients of her services are rewarded by success will possibly see little need to weigh the implications of the divergence of professional imperatives from agency norms. The worker whose efforts fail, however, may be less sanguine about operational norms. Consider, for example, the following report about the operational norm of a social service agency, which is based on hearings held by the United States Senate Public Works Subcommittee investigating disaster relief agencies in the aftermath of a hurricane:

> The major issue, particularly in the case of the Red Cross, is whether relief should be distributed on the basis of predisaster economic status, or whether it should be granted strictly on the basis of individual need and the establishment of minimum standards of adequacy for all disaster victims.
> The Red Cross manual for assistance to disaster victims is steeped in the doctrine that they be restored to normalcy; that they should

receive aid in proportion to the standard of living to which they were previously accustomed.

On the surface this position sounds eminently fair to most middle-class Americans but to many Negroes it is another manifestation of a white-oriented society, the black leaders testified.

The point the Negroes raised is basically this: what is the value of returning a family to their pre-hurricane status when that condition was already one of wretchedness? The Negro mother needing clothing for her children is angry and bitter when she is given second-hand goods while the middle-class mother is issued new clothing, they said.

There is little consolation for the Negro who remains in a tar-papered shack and watches the Red Cross pay for the construction of a new home for his white employer, the black leader argued.[17]

The aftermath of a sudden catastrophe like the hurricane in question can highlight the consistent way in which earlier inequalities beget later ones. For the worker called upon to administer the services of an agency, the contradictions between agency and professional imperatives can be dramatic. Both the subtle and the obvious shortcomings of a program will be evident not only to those shortchanged by it but also to those whose work keeps them in close touch with its consequences.

A number of options are conceivably open to a worker faced with conflicting directives; and if the commendations imposed by that part of the community responsible for allocating resources to the agency are accepted as good and sound, an effort must be made to reconcile professional imperatives to these commendations.

The rules governing agency operational norms are not derived from principle commendations that conflict with such norms. A not uncommon option is thus to treat every such rule as an independent command and isolate it from all others. As was noted earlier, the formulation of each rule

17. John A. Nordheimer, "U.S. Disaster Relief and Built-in Bias," *New York Times,* reprinted in *San Francisco Chronicle,* January 13, 1970.

gives neither the commendation nor the proposition that justifies it. Each rule can therefore be treated independently without altering either the command or the tasks essential to its implementation. As a consequence of this option, the work is reduced to an efficient mechanical routine that keeps worker choices and judgments to a minimum—an instance of 'simply carrying out orders.'

Under a second option, the practice principle is treated as a propositional statement only and its commendative aspect is ignored. The principle then becomes a morally neutral knowledge directive, and the resulting practice is judged by its efficiency because in respect to this principle it is without any goal. It is assumed that although the professional worker makes his skills available to society, she can be responsible neither for the uses to which they are put nor for those consequences that are beyond her ability or right to control. A modified version of this option requires the worker to assume that the commendation in the practice principle is in fact a 'know that' truth. Here again the principle is reduced to a propositional statement.

Under yet a third option, the imperatives implicit in the operational norm are treated as a competing set at odds with those of the profession. This conflict is then considered as a necessary reflection of a "realistic" view of how things work in society. Under these circumstances, the points at issue must be decided by the competition in the marketplace of ideals rather than the worker. Meanwhile, the worker, as an employee of the agency, must abide by current agency norms.[18]

There are probably other options. All share the requirement that the worker believe that she is responsible neither for the conflict identified nor for its resolution and that the conflict is not significant or relevant to her practice. If this

18. Harold Lewis, "The Battered Helper," *Child Welfare* 59, no. 4 (April 1980): 195–201.

analysis of options has merit, one is forced to conclude that those workers who take their profession's ethical imperatives most seriously will also be most reluctant to choose any of these options in value conflict situations. They would be more likely to challenge the practices, policies, and programs based on conflicting norms. Such workers may prove to be the heretics on the staffs of social agencies. They may also prove to be the most precious resource of the profession — leading efforts to right community wrongs and to correct distributive injustices. A profession ought to cultivate such a resource, provide moral sanction for the efforts of such workers, and not confuse them with the irresponsible and the self-seeking.

»»   ««

In this chapter as in Chapter 7, I consider how knowledge and values contribute to practice. It is now possible to bring the analysis of work and that of the worker together in the light of what has been revealed about rules, principles, theory, ethics, knowledge, and values. Happily, all these elements jointly contribute to that attribute so much sought and cherished — skill. To introduce an analysis of skill, I must first attend to what gives skill its attractions — style.

CHAPTER EIGHT

»» ««

Style

THE INTELLECTUAL TOOLS we have considered all facilitate the mental work required for an informed and purposeful professional practice. Style also facilitates such work; but in its most significant attributes, it differs from the tools we have described. Style encapsulates no observations for storage in memory to be recovered for use in practice. Instead, style endows a practice with its attractions and in so doing adds an enriching ingredient to skill. Because style is sometimes equated with skill, practice is sometimes mistaken for art. This is unfortunate but understandable.

As a form of assembling, style exhibits the manner in which each person arranges what she apprehends in her actions and their product.[1] Identical styles may be as rare as identical physiques; but like physiques, styles both help to identify individuals and permit the classification of types. The persistence of personal, professional, recipient, and agency styles suggests that style can and should be evaluated. We may come to know about style as it impinges upon practice in the same sense that we come to know about anything else that impinges on practice. A theory of practice cannot be complete unless it accounts for style.

1. Meyer Shapiro, "Style," in *Anthropology Today,* ed. Al Krocker (Berkeley and Los Angeles: University of California Press, 1953), pp. 287–312.

The complexity of the process by which principles ultimately shape a product can be attributed to the fact that principles do not in their prior state resemble their manifestation in the product.[2] The necessity that a principle be translated into rules before it can be applied in a way that fulfills the conditions set by the principle opens the process to a wide range of influences—including the styles of practitioners, agencies, and the profession. Practice thus imparts great variety to the form of the product as it is shaped by the application of rules actually intended to translate the same principle consistently to the same service situation. The practitioner's freedom to translate in her own way assures a recognizable uniformity in the product not governed by prescribed methods, and this uniformity communicates the art of individual practice to the product.

Methods that seek to impart a preferred order to a process assume the existence of an order that has to be altered or a disorder that has to be arranged. As I have noted, if differences in the product resulting from the influence of styles in the application of rules are to be distinguished from simple disorder or from inappropriate order, some criteria are necessary for recognizing stylistic differences as well as methodological.

Consider the following description of a personal style:

"She just sat there, looking into me, and said nothing." I recall the anguish with which my classmate reported to the nervous, attentive listeners her agonizing conference with her faculty advisor. Once before, she had received a reminder note, that a conference with the advisor was overdue. She had dutifully arranged her appointment, though she couldn't think if a good reason for going, nor guess at the reason she was beckoned. The first conference turned into a nightmare. The advisor had greeted her with a nod and a smile, directing her to a chair beside the desk at which she

2. Justus Buchler, *The Concept of Method* (New York: Columbia University Press, 1961), p. 4.

was seated. And then nothing, not a word. My classmate did not know where or when to begin, nor what to talk about. After five minutes of silence, a terror took hold of her and she managed to wonder out loud, "What is it you wanted to see me about?" The response, totally unexpected and unbelievable, "This is your hour, how do you want to use it?" left her dumbfounded. After another two minutes of silence, she felt she had to get out and away, or she would scream, and she simply stood up, thanked her advisor and left. Two days later, another note, and this second conference. And, as she said of her advisor, "She just sat there, looking into me, and said nothing." This time, after a minute of silence, my class-mate asked, "Is there something wrong in what I've been doing that you want to share with me?" And again the answer, "This is your hour, how do you want to use it?" For most of those listening, this second report confirmed their worst fears. This advisor was a "character," and despite her national reputation as a practitioner and theoretician, survival in the School was contingent on avoiding close contact with her. It was certain death to have her as an advisor.

I didn't understand what was really troubling my classmate, for the anguish I detected was more a self-evaluation than a reaction to an outside criticism. I finally got her alone, away from the dining room table where all the students and staff living at the Settlement shared our family-type meals, and asked her what was so upsetting. After all, the reported incident was predictable, given the exper-ience of others before her. She preferred not to talk about it, but bathed me in tears instead. After the sobbing let up, she dropped all pretext of control and poured out all the fears, failures, and hopelessness that inadequate efforts at helping had stored up in her, ending with the anguished tone—"And she saw it all in me, including my determination not to ask for help, but to manage it all on my own. She looked *in* me, and saw it all. She didn't have to say a word, she left out everything except what was absolutely necessary for me to have if *I* wanted to take help. She had arranged the conference, she had not imposed an agenda; she had been totally available to me, and she had repeated the offer after my first resistance to her way of saying, 'I'm here for you to use me.' She saw *in me*; she understood what was bothering me; and she asked me to chose between the pain of my inner doubts or the pain I felt in having to admit I needed help, if I was going to learn to give it."

This advisor, whom I got to know as well as most students get to know their professors, had *style*. In appearance unimposing, she was in her active fifties, and not too well, physically. Possibly, a thyroid condition caused her eyes to bulge outward. They captured your attention at first contact, and locked you into their orbit until a blink broke the contact, or her head turned to release you from their control. Never, or almost never, did you initiate closure, even if at times you wished to pull away to cover the nakedness you felt in her presence. This advisor, whom the student experienced in her silence, also had a talent for the concise, perceptive, clear, and what Suzanne Langer calls the presentational when she spoke. Images captured in a phrase; full arguments launched and concluded in few words, all carefully selected and appropriate. One did not relate to her, one engaged with her; and never a superficial engagement at that. When she shared her troubles and doubts; when she pinpointed the humor in a desperate situation; when she asserted strongly held beliefs and deeply felt convictions without discrediting your own, the same style came through. It reached the point where I could perceive in secondary sources a comment as her's; could guess when her point of view was being presented; could even even predict what would upset or please her in someone else's class paper. Her style was so powerfully formed and richly embellished, its distinctive flavor and color were recognizable even when not immediately related to her person.[3]

As this illustration suggests, style is a consistent arrangement and sequence of elements in a process that imparts to an action or product an unmistakable identity. In professional practices where styles are manifest more in action than in a product (teaching, for example, in contrast to architecture), the opportunity to hear or observe the style is curtailed; and one must often depend on records or secondary reports to learn the peculiarities of a distinctive style. This factor, however, in no way belittles the role of style in

3. Harold Lewis, "Style in Professional Practice," unpublished paper, Hunter College School of Social Work, New York, 1975; see Jacob Fisher, *The Response of Social Work to the Depression* (Cambridge, Mass.: Schenkman Publishing Co., 1980), p. 83, for another description of the teacher described in Lewis's paper.

teaching — as every student knows. All professions, moreover, have their own styles, as unique as personal styles. Although these professional styles change over the years, one can decipher dominant professional styles in different periods. Organizations also cultivate and display distinctive styles through their logos, offices, programs, staffing patterns, and the like. The vault like appearance of the bank exudes a sense of security. The use of the vernacular in prayer conveys to parishioners the relevance of doctrine to the here and now. The conservative Republican high collar of the Hoover administration gave way to the Liberal Democratic hat and elevated cigarette holder of the Roosevelt era. The messages communicated through style are of such significance that as much concern is often attached to its absence as is given its distinctive presence. Told that President Coolidge had died, Alice Roosevelt Longworth asked, "How can they tell?"

Personal style asserts the individuality and consistency of its creator. In the performance of a task, a worker focuses her attention on the application of prescribed guidelines to appropriate, timely, consistent, and uniform behavior.[4] A worker may be peripherally aware of the seemingly irrelevant accompaniments of her task; but when these irrelevancies begin to command more of the worker's attention, they often begin to distract her so much that her practice becomes clumsy or stops entirely. The same kind of thing happens when one ends a phone conversation abruptly because one notices the flashing light that says another caller has been put on hold. When the worker rearranges these distractions into some new order, they may compete for her attention with the prescribed guidelines and paralyze her action. This happens in practice when extraordinary actions displace expected behaviors. A normal facial expression, for example, becomes

4. Michael Polanyi, *Personal Knowledge* (Chicago: University of Chicago Press, 1958), pp. 55–56.

a tic or an inappropriate grimace. In positive circumstances, when the arrangement can be integrated with the associated prescribed behavior, an innovative practice results—a practice that reflects a distinctive style.[5] Different capacities for arranging disparate subsidiary awarenesses in relation to focal awareness reflect different talents that are evident in the different styles of skill that result from their application. It may have been a serendipitous insight of Archimedes that led him to cry out "Eureka," but it is unique to Archimedes' style that he consistently experienced such insights during his lifetime.

Thus, the hallmark of style is its possessor's consistent and persistent ability to make connections between subsidiary awareness and focal awareness. Where lack of opportunity restricts a practitioner's willingness or capacity to pursue such connections and where the practitioner herself lacks the ability to make them, the style evidenced in the practice of prescribed actions will most likely be less personal—shaped by the agency's and the profession's formalized style and codified into rule-governed guidelines.

When the changes influenced by individual styles are communicated to a substantial number of practitioners, they can modify the esthetics of practice and enrich its attractions. If they are then generalized to govern an area of practice, radical innovations in style can also revolutionize methods of practice. Illustrations of these phenomena readily come to mind: the dress, appearance, language, and use of time of the settlement-house detached gang worker contrast sharply with those of the office-based counselor practicing psychotherapy. The white coat of the hospital social worker, the uniform of the army social worker, the dungarees of the camp social worker—each conveys an institutional style, even as personal attributes like hair style and other niceties (including how each wears the uniform) may mark distinctive personal styles.

5. Erving Goffman, *Encounters* (Indianapolis: Bobbs-Merrill, 1961) p. 45, 55, 151.

In the case of the social work educator whose style prompted the thumbnail sketch quoted earlier, she certainly held to her school's style in scheduling advisee contacts; in holding the interview in her office rather than an elevator or corridor; in limiting the time to an hour; and in divers other ways. Her behavior during the student conference also evidenced a professional style not uncommon in those days when theory justified the "passive approach." Nevertheless, neither the school as an institution, nor the theoretical justifications of the profession determined her unique use of eye contact, her masterful use of language and movement, her insightful, razor-sharp written comments on papers, and her unswerving willingness to engage deeply in the helping relationship. On the contrary, many students began to mimic her style in their contact with clients — with varying degrees of success. Unlike most other professors, she communicated a distinctive personal style so attractive that her students wanted to adopt it in shaping their methods of work.[6] To judge from her style, such emulation was probably contrary to her intention. More than most others, she cherished and encouraged the richness of divergent personal styles so long as she thought they incorporated agency and professional styles and did not detract from the service to which each client was entitled.

A student's efforts to mimic her teacher's style and the teacher's encouragement of students to enrich their individual styles both suggest assumptions about the nature and origin of styles that deserve more attention than is normally given to them. Students behave as though styles can be acquired; teachers as though styles are a given, perhaps at birth. Obviously, these are not either/or possibilities.

6. John D. Ingalls, *A Trainer's Guide to Andragogy: An Artistic Approach to Educational Design* (Washington, D.C.: U.S. Department of Health, Education and Welfare, 1972), p. 54, suggests the challenge to the educator to design a learning experience both artistically and esthetically satisfying to the learner.

Consider the six-year-old who, upon being introduced to a tomato growing on its vine, remarks, "This is a nice plant, but it has bad posture." When this same six-year-old, hearing Eliza Dolittle's language from a recording of *My Fair Lady,* explains to a friend, "She talks crooked and he straightens her out," one is inclined to think that this child's unique formulations are located in unique sensitivities he brought with him into the world. Poincaré believed that his study of the history of mathematics supported the hypothesis that analytical styles were primarily responsible for discoveries in the algebras while gestalt types were primarily responsible for discoveries in the geometries.[7] In terms of current brain research, he would be ascribing to right or left hemisphere development, the particular style of the innovator in mathematics.[8] Stressing cultural influences, Edward Hall described the stances and postures of nationality types during conversations so clearly that one could with relative certainty recognize an American with his hands in his pockets and his slouched informality; the German with his formal stiffness, bending at the hip; the Italian standing at a distance and waving his arms.[9] Others have noted that urban types tend to be interested in what is manufactured rather than what grows; in what is invented rather than what is discovered; in what is predictable rather than what develops.

7. Henri Poincaré, *Science et méthode* (Paris, 1908), includes this essay on the genesis of mathematical creation.

8. For example, see Nigel Calder, *The Mind of Man* (New York: Viking Press, 1970), pp. 243–52.

9. Edward Hall, *The Silent Language* (New York: Doubleday, 1959), pp. 187–209; see also Shirley Weitz, ed., *Nonverbal Communication* (New York: Oxford University Press, 1974), pp. 127–99; Albert E. Schefflin, *How Behavior Means* (New York: Jason Aronson, 1974), pp. 97–116; Edmund Leach, "The Influence of Cultural Context on Non-Verbal Communication in Man," in *Non-Verbal Communication,* ed. R.A. Hinde (Cambridge: At the University Press, 1972), pp. 315–43.

They have contrasted this urban style with the rural type, for whom natural processes hold a greater attraction. We need not elaborate on examples that explain either the genetic or the cultural origins of styles.[10] There is ample evidence that both are involved in the evolution of a style; and both must be considered in any effort to understand and enrich professional and agency styles through the appropriate utilization of personal styles.

Perhaps one approach to the matter of developing and utilizing styles is to examine the styles people use when they ask questions.[11] If one systematically observes people formulating questions, one soon identifies two predominant styles—and a lesser number of people characterized by their unusual use of both. Some people formulate questions in global terms, investing each question with so much feeling that one can hardly modify it without threatening the significance its maker attributes to it. Thus, a young mother overwhelmed by the stress brought on by an alcoholic husband, two preschool children, a full-time job, and a chronic state of physical exhaustion tells the worker she's ready to give up, just forget about work, and confine herself to maintaining the home. To this total proposition, the worker who also thinks globally responds with the question, "Do you really want to give up, with all that would entail?" If you suggested to the worker that the question is too all-encompassing for the mother to handle, she will respond "It is her question, it is the central question; it cannot be ignored and must be con-

10. Alan Lomax, "The Evolution of Culture and Expressive Style: A Comparative Approach to Social Change," in *Social Change and Human Behavior,* ed. George V. Coelho and Eli A. Rubenstein, (Rockville, Maryland: National Institute of Mental Health, 1972), pp. 41–67.

11. Harold Lewis, "The Significance for Social Work Education of the Student's Approach to the Formulation of a Research Question," *Social Work Education Reporter* 9, no. 2 (April 1961).

fronted." Another worker who thinks more analytically, might decide that the totality of the stated problem might itself possibly be the most serious problem and that it could be helpful if the issues were dealt with discretely. She could formulate her question, possibly in relation to how the children were posing problems, turning this issue into a focal point from which the whole could be placed in perspective.

In an actual case, a mother said breakfast set the tone for the whole day. Her younger daughter swallowed a whole glass of orange juice in one gigantic gurgling gulp. The mother tried to stop her by pulling the glass away from her lips. The inevitable screaming, tantrums, and tears followed, upsetting the older child and ruining the start of the day for all three. The worker asked the mother if she had tried putting just enough juice into the glass for what she considered a one-gulp portion, then adding another and another until the juice was finished. The mother had not but would try. The next week, still complaining, she interrupted her critical outpouring with a sudden smile, and for the first cheerful note in months, reported, "You know, that suggestion about the juice worked—no fights around that for the whole week."

Global styles are more productive and fruitful in helping relationships when those who have them learn to break totalities down into their components. Without yielding their concern for the whole, such helpers direct the client to see the whole in a part that may not be as overwhelming and to work on that. The analytic style, on the other hand, can profit from a technique that calls for less control and permits more risk in the helping relationship. In neither case will personal style be sacrificed; but in both cases, the clientele—whatever their styles—have greater opportunities to utilize their own idiosyncratic styles with more support and less constraint.

Another significant dimension of style can be seen in the way organizations, professions, and individuals use time. When the way students use time to carry out research theses was systematically monitored, a startling finding showed the significant and distinctive influence of style on both work patterns and perception of time.[12] The students prepared weekly schedules throughout the semester as they worked on and completed their theses. Each schedule asked for the following information: What was worked on? When? For how long? In what location? Schedules were collected each week and by end of the semester all theses were completed. Two weeks after the next semester began, all students who had completed theses the previous semester, including those observed, filled out schedules that asked them to make judgments about their use of time while working on their theses the previous term. What tasks took the longest time? Where was most of the work done? During what times of day was most work done? The final question asked them to guess whether they had spent more, less, or about the same amount of time on their theses, than had their classmates. In addition, the faculty was asked to rank all students included in the survey in overall ability, but this faculty judgment was not related to where, when, or what tasks the students worked on longest. Bizarre use of time was associated with students judged to be emotionally upset, but too few cases occurred to warrant any generalizations. The startling finding, which appeared to separate the students judged most able from those judged weakest, was their own judgments about their use of time in comparison to that of their classmates. The ablest students uniformly believed they had spent more time on their theses than had others—despite the fact that their self-reports showed no such pattern. The weakest students thought they had spent less time, or about the same time as others, though the data did not support

12. Harold Lewis, "Students' Use of Time in Completing Master's Degree Research Projects," unpublished paper, University of Pennsylvania School of Social Work, Philadelphia, 1960.

these impressions either. From discussions with the students, it became evident that the able students felt they had to sacrifice many other uses of time to complete their theses, while the weak students hardly ever raised this issue. One practical use of this finding was that it ended the annual bout of faculty soul searching brought on by student complaints about the inordinate amount of time spent on theses. A quick check of complainers identified few indeed whose actual time spent related to the complaint in any way. For example, one student, who had spent the least time of any (a good student), complained that the theses took too long, while another, who had spent by far the most time, (also a good student), thought she had not spent much time, (nor enough time) on her thesis.

In *The Silent Language,* Edward Hall devotes considerable detailed attention to the formal, informal, and technical meanings of time as significant dimensions that impart distinctive styles to a culture.[13] Any professional working for an institution quickly learns that institution's *time* expectations. Of the twenty-eight definitions of time cited in *Webster's International Dictionary,* some direct our attention to the genetic, biological, and internal timing organs while others focus our attention on the external and cultural time patterns.[14]

>> <<

Even a cursory review of our professional literature highlights how little has been done to study and understand the influence of style on skill. With the exception of Jessie Tafts's

13. Hall, *Silent Language,* pp. 165–85.
14. See "Biological Rhythms in Psychiatry and Medicine," (Bethesda, Md.: National Institute of Mental Health, National Clearing House for Mental Health Information, 1970).

seminal essay, even less has been done on the influence of time in promoting the creativity inherent in a worker's style.[15] When we look back at the description of one teacher's style given, we can now note how she exercised influence by setting time-limits (the available hour); by using periodic reinforcement (the second request for a conference coming shortly after the first); by intensifying the meaning of time (prolonged, unexpected silence); by promptly initiating the request for a conference (the student's failure to make contact in due time, which presumably served as a warning of some difficulty to be pursued); by agitating the student's feeling of inner clock time (I couldn't stand it any longer; I had to get away); and by implying to the student that within the constraints of the available time (the semester) she was out-of-step and would run out of time unless something changed. That she utilized so many facets of time in a manner consistent with the other dimensions of her powerful style is evidence of her considerable talent. Unfortunately, the social work profession has not explored the significance of style in skill and has not become prepared to evaluate it. We neverthless rush on to determine competence, which in good measure is based on skill.

It is no longer sufficient to describe professional practice as an art that utilizes science in the service of those seeking help. The art needs to be explicated, so that skill in practice need not be confused only with its attractions. The art of practice is to be found neither in the worker nor in the client, but in the product of their relationship; and in that relationship, the distinctive styles of the worker and client coalesce to give each helping transaction its unique, idiosyncratic attri-

15. Jessie Taft, *The Dynamics of Therapy in a Controlled Relationship,* 2d ed. (New York: Dover Books, 1962), pp. 3–23.

butes.[16] Until we know more than we now do about the role of style in the helping relationship, we will make little progress toward the demystification of that relationship and little that permits it to be viewed as a fully observable and knowable experience.

16. Ruth H. Lebovitz, "An Inquiry into the Nature of Change in Casework Helping through an Examination of the Art Element in Casework Practice" (D.S.W. diss., University of Pennsylvania, 1968).

»» ««

CHAPTER NINE

Skill

W HEN WORK IS WELL DONE, it is usually appreciated for its skill. For the worker whose self-respect is invested in her work, to be judged skillful is a matter for pride. Besides, promotion, recognition, status, and other benefits are likely to follow when the judgment is made by those she works for or by peers engaged in similar work. Although there is agreement that skill appears in the work of different practitioners in a manner that permits comparison, efforts to grade practitioners in relation to skill have recognized the exacting, often unrewarding results associated with such judgments. Because skill incorporates all the elements of work discussed thus far, it can be used to examine their relationships to each other and to the skillful act itself. Table 2 depicts these relationships in a simplified form.

A worker judges skill by evaluating the work done. She recognizes from experience that skill in social work is directly observable in the act rather than the actor or the product.

The essentials of skill must be understood in concert with one other.[1] References to "knowledge and skill," or "knowledge, values, and skill," which are common in the literature, support the misleading notion that skill itself does

1. Michael Polanyi, *Personal Knowledge* (Chicago: University of Chicago Press, 1958).

Table 2. Diagrammatic Evaluation of Degrees of Skill

Degree of Skill	Dimensions of Skill			
	Knowledge	Action	Values	Style
Advanced professional (expert)	Theories	Design	Ethical imperatives	Personal, professional, and agency
Professional (master)	Propositions	Method	Commendations	Professional and agency
Preprofessional (technician)	Directives	Technique/ tool	Commands	Agency

not encompass knowledge and values. An unfortunate by-product of this erroneous view is the pervasive belief that the cognitive and the emotive are separable in both the act and the actors. Some writers have gone so far as to argue that different types inhabit the profession: the researchers (scientific types who do the thinking) and the artists (imaginative types who do the feeling).[2] Such misleading formulations are costly to the profession: They retard the development of sound education for practice.

There is consensus among those who write about it that skill is informed, and therefore knowledge based, and that skill is also manifest in action requiring the implementation of a method or procedure. There is less agreement that skill is intentioned, and therefore value laden, or that it is idiosyncratic, bearing the attraction of institutional, professional, and individual styles. We assume that knowledge, action, values, and style are essential dimensions of skill and therefore need to be understood jointly. In the following discus-

2. Margaret Blenkner, "Obstacles for Evaluative Research in Casework," *Social Casework* 31, no. 2 (February 1950): 56.

sion, these dimensions are considered in detail not only to provide a substantive view of the content of skill but also to elicit some measure for judging degrees of skill.

KNOWLEDGE

UNINFORMED PRACTICE is usually characterized by unsystematic, unpredictable behavior in which chance plays a major role in accounting for whatever results are achieved. Sustained effort is justified by faith and fate; and fact and fiction are indistinguishable in the practitioner's report on what works or does not work and why. If you ask a worker what led her to do what she did, and she cites intuition, insight, and the signs of the zodiac as reasons, you have cause for concern.[3] Both theory and reasoned association between the known and the expected are alien to this worker. Unlike the skilled practitioner who entertains a hypothesis even when she is uncertain of its truth, the uninformed worker entertains none and often accepts logically indefensible propositions as truths. For an unskilled worker, certainty often represents the right to be wrong at the top of her voice.

It is not necessary for practitioners to be equally knowing to assure equally useful practices. Either a caseworker supervisor or a case aide, for example, can equally help a recipient complete an application for homemaker services. If each follows the rules that assure appropriate action in a well-defined request for help, a systematic and predictable behavior should follow. Such rules help to generate habituated behavior in the worker who applies them because they can be followed with minimal personal judgment. For this reason, technolo-

3. See Martin Bloom, *The Paradox of Helping: Introduction to the Philosophy of Scientific Practice* (New York: John Wiley & Sons, 1975), pp. 53–67.

gies that contain a great amount of skillful practice nevertheless require little professional judgment and therefore demand minimal skill in their application. When her behavior is prescribed, it is unnecessary for a practitioner to be professionally informed. Under such circumstances, the decision to use the technology—not the application of the technique itself—demands professional skill. Knowing how to use the phone and knowing when to use it both involve judgments, but the two are of a different order. Knowing how to respond to phone calls in a suicide prevention center involves judgments of a different order from those needed in answering inquiries about agency services.

In complex judgments, four different levels of intellectual demand can be required. At the simplest level (for example, when a program aide assigns children to seats in a day-care center bus), a rule can be followed with few requirements for worker judgment. At the next level (assigning workloads to professional staff, for example) a choice must be made among rules, and relevant propositions that anticipate the consequences must inform the choice. At the third level (say, allocating limited resources to competing programs) the task requires a choice among propositions and it is desirable to have some understanding of the theory or theories that can place these propositions and their related programs in some sequence of priorities. At the highest level (choosing among psychodynamic, behavioral, and existential modes of helping as the methods of choice for an agency's practice) it is necessary to choose among theories, and an understanding of what is known but not explained by a particular theory (as well as what is known and explained by alternative theories) is essential. In brief, degrees of complexity in judgment can be determined by the type of intellectual effort required.

We can differentiate the intellectual work further if we consider the reasoning that such work entails. For example, when routine activities are required—when a worker identifies, describes, and classifies a range of evidence that meets the legal definition of neglect—the task calls for an enumeration of alternatives from which choices will be made. The worker is expected to list what can be ascertained and include all known possibilities. When no clear routine is evident and propositions are required to inform the activities, the worker is expected to arrange the alternatives along some scale of priorities.

In cases of child neglect, a worker must rank the alternatives that might provide protection for the child and assist the family in changing its neglectful behavior. To perform this task, the worker must conceive of appropriate criteria for ordering choices, weight the criteria on the basis of the available evidence and sequence the alternatives, recognize and take into account the intercorrelations that influence the sequence of alternatives, and finally, anticipate the probable changes in priorities that would follow their implementation. In addition to identification, description, and classification, the worker's equipment must include a grasp of typologies, some knowledge of the alternatives for intervention, and an ability to scale the mix of both the typologies of conditions deemed neglectful and the types of intervention deemed appropriate. Thus far, she will undoubtedly have identified neglect and possibly classified it into one of three major categories—physical, emotional, or supervisory.

The worker may also have classified the options for action that will protect the child to include one of the following in addition to counseling: *(1)* providing a homemaker; *(2)* removing the child to the custody of a competent relative; *(3)* placing the child in a temporary shelter; or *(4)* remanding the child to the custody of the court to assure appropriate supervision. Weighting the areas of neglect and the various care arrangements, the worker may feel that the fourth alternative is the only one likely to effect a change in the child's situation. But if that option is not available, options two, three, and one—in that order—should be pursued. Having finally chosen the order, the worker decides to act on the options in the order specified. Besides explaining how this particular intervention will yield the desired result, her decision will require certain ancillary information—knowledge of the status of the court calendar, of the attitude of the sitting judge, of the alternatives available to the court—all the elements that influence the chance that the court will support a judgment of neglect requiring removal.

Although the worker's decision to act is informed by judgments, even more is required. She must believe that her judgments have produced the basis for a decision. She must conclude that the moment for decision has arrived because all possible evidence has been considered and the decision is both timely and appropriate. Obviously, such a decision cannot be made without relating action to the wider setting of practice.

In addition to intellectual factors, other issues contribute to the complexity of situations requiring judgment. For example, the completeness of the information, the mood and temper of the person making the judgment, and the environment in which the judgment is made all increase the difficulty of arriving at sound judgments. It remains essential, however, that difficulty in making judgments not be confused with the intrinsic complexity of those judgments. It is possible for both the simplest judgments and the most complex to encounter similar difficulties. Nevertheless, under normal conditions, the level of practice skill is judged in part by the cognitive ability required properly to inform the practice.

ACTION

TECHNIQUE is the aspect of skill necessary for action. Technique provides the worker with an orderly procedure for accomplishing a desired aim. Knowing 'what' and 'where' may orient the worker to the tasks; but without mastery of the 'how' of implementation, she will not bring the performance off. Like the electronics theorist who cannot repair his own stereo set, the scholar who knows all about helping and theories of helping may be better at receiving help than at giving it.

Related sets of techniques collectively make up methods. Methods acculturate the practitioner to the profession and its practice in a pervasive and fundamental way; they also transmit to action the accumulated and tested wisdom of the past. Every technical tool represents the investment of years of experience, experiment, discovery, and invention. To the novice (who may be totally unaware of this investment), an agency admission form may impart a level of methodological sophistication she could hardly achieve so rapidly and accurately from any other learning opportunity.

This technical power of method is often attractive to those looking for facile solutions to difficult problems in uncertain situations. For example, what I call the checklist syndrome — listing and totaling of problems as a magic substitute for assessment — has developed in recent years; but the professional skills associated with action in uncertain situations do not lie in such techniques. Rather, a skilled professional must master techniques in order to utilize appropriate methods in the design of a program of intervention.

Tools useful for technical work take many forms: physical, mental, emotional, or any combination of the three. A technical tool can be as ordinary as a checklist or a registration card or as complex as a computer, a calculus, or a high level of self-awareness. Neither the form of a tool nor the difficulty of its use marks its user as a professional. It is the judgment entailed in the design and application of the technique that use these tools that truly shows action skills.

A practice deficient in technical tools tends to be more dependent on professional judgments. The advent of sophisticated drugs and complex diagnostic instruments has created a number of technical specialties in medicine and opened up to nonmedical personnel many tasks formerly seen as a doctor's alone. Although fewer technical advances have been achieved in social work, more is becoming known about the administrative, relational, and learning elements of the helping methods used by the profession; and social workers can expect that as important technologies develop technicians will perform many of the tasks currently calling for professional decisions.

INTENTIONS AND VALUES

THAT SKILL implies intent is evident in what is favored or disfavored in its application. When a worker engages in some sensible action, she is trying to realize something worthwhile or avoid something undesirable. For example, she removes a child from a threatening home situation both to provide a more caring milieu and to avoid the dangers to which he would otherwise be exposed. A problem can be created, however, when the worker's intentions fail to appear in the product of her work. Substitute care or care in an institution, for example, may ultimately be more damaging to the child than his own home. In social work practice, an ability to avoid this separation of intent and result is an important measure of professional skill.

In her practice, therefore, a skilled practitioner will act so as to assure that the intent of the service she provides is informed by values. Such a practitioner both knows and communicates the ethical imperatives that guide her intentions. She can enumerate the oughts, shoulds, musts, and shalls that circumscribe the permissible limits to innovation and creativity as she seeks to realize the consequences she wants from her efforts. In addition, such a worker shows her ability to imagine and apply unique and original responses to requests for service; she will continuously explore the 'possible' contained within the constraints of the ethical.

We must assume that the recipients of service bring their own intentions to contacts with workers. Part of professional skill is evident in a worker's capacity for incorporating recipients' expectations into the intention that guides her practice. When these resources and actions for service apply to an institution, a similar requirement holds for its organizational expectations. Obviously, the worker's tasks will vary in complexity as she seeks to assure that her service is informed by values. These variations can serve as a value-related measure of the degree of skill present in practice.

At the simplest level, when the worker is simply following rule-governed directives, no value component seems to be involved. For example, instructions to clear with a social service exchange; to ask for the names of other agencies or professional persons helping with the need identified; or to note all sources of the recipient's support, financial or otherwise, do not carry any clear intention other than that of gathering information. What is overlooked in such activities is the commanding nature of the rule, in addition to its simple directive. That you shall (must, will) do these things is implicit in each instruction. When the practitioner seeks the justification for the command, she will not find it in the if–then propositions that inform the directives. As noted earlier, the justification is located in an ethical imperative related to some fundamental value that underpins the goals of the service.

Thus at the more complex level, when principles of practice combine a proposition based in theory with a commendation justified by ethics, the judgment required of workers is more difficult. The instructions cited in the preceding paragraph, for example, could be taken to suggest the principle that efforts on a recipient's behalf should be coordinated to maximize their benefits. Certainly, each of these instructions could assist in such coordination. In fact, many other rule-type directives could be analyzed to find the intention embedded in this principle. On the other hand, the same set of instructions could be taken to fulfill the opposite intention — that recipients will be discouraged from exploiting limited resources unfairly if the worker determines whether duplication of services is involved.

It is not possible to determine which of these intentions (if not both) is being implemented in the worker's behavior without identifying the relevant ethical guideline. Thus, if the value sought is justice, and if the ethical imperative requires that unequal advantage in the provision of service is justified only if such advantage raises both the expectations and the resources available for the most disadvantaged recipients, the shoulds, musts, and shalls would support efforts intended to achieve coordination so as to maximize what is available — particularly for those least able to manage the agency service network on their own — and thereby avoid inequities generated by the service system itself.[4]

The ways an ethic may be implemented are limited only by resources and imagination, and the more skilled worker draws on both in formulating practice principles. She will then use these principles to assure adherence to the intentions prescribed by the ethic. Practice sometimes generates value dilemmas, for which there are no ethical prescriptions. In such instances, considerable axiological skill is required to develop an adequate ethical framework.

What laws are to science, ethical prescriptions are to values: They orient the worker to the essentials that delineate the values inherent in application. The worker cannot violate ethical prescriptions in practice without departing from the values used to justify the goals of her actions. We have previously considered what is involved in the formulation of such prescrip-

4. John Rawls, *A Theory of Justice* (Cambridge: Harvard University Press, Belknap Press, 1971).

tions, what is required in their appropriate application to the development of practice principles, and what is expected in following their guidelines in the provision of service. All entail skill, but this skill decreases as the level of complexity decreases.

STYLE

STYLE AS AN element of skill will be evident in both the performance and the product of the professional activity. Adept or inept, adroit or awkward, deft or clumsy, the style of the practitioner will be characterized by its attractions, not by the values and knowledge that inform it. The beauty (or lack of beauty) of the product—the simplicity, coherence, clarity, precision, balance, and harmony it shows—will attest to the practitioner's style, not to the product's rightness or goodness. Inevitably, style transmits the warmth and color of the human involvement in the helping process. Those who mistake style for all of skill—who fail to appreciate the values and knowledge that in fact constitute its essence—confuse skill with intuitive art.

The first observation to be made about style is also the most crucial: Both a task that requires limited skill and a task that requires considerable skill can be performed attractively, even beautifully. The degree of skill required does not vary in proportion to the style with which it is carried out; in other words, style (unlike the other dimensions of skill) cannot be used to measure degree of skill. Those so confused as to think otherwise will subject recipients to great risks. Helping an unwed mother decide whether to keep her child or relinquish it requires considerable skill, even if the process is ill devised and lacking in refinement; helping the mother to choose a maternity wardrobe within the limits of her means requires less skill, even if it is done with unusual grace and sophistication. The judgments entailed in each of these tasks need not be informed to the same degree—the ethical and cognitive issues are of a different order, and the choices to be made are qualitatively different in their demands upon the practitioner.

In addition, the idiosyncratic elements of style need discipline. Having to manage not only agency and professional styles but also the elements of style that shape the activities of the service recipient, the worker must scrupulously control her personal style without sacrificing its unique and enhancing attributes.

Like all the other elements of skill, styles change over time. Many influences, including natural maturation, alter a practitioner's style. Those attributes unique to a particular style nevertheless are likely to remain visible in the idiosyncratic thread that marks the work of its creator. This quality of style—the consistent survival of the traits by which it is identified despite changes in the elements that form it—makes style identifiable at different times and in different contexts.

There are limits to the variations in style tolerable in any one setting. A style particularly appropriate in one form of practice can be highly inappropriate in another. Post-mortem reviews to determine why some well-informed, principled, and methodologically proficient person could not make it in a particular organization occasionally highlight this problematic aspect of style. Of all the attributes of skill, style alone asserts the individuality of the practitioner in a fashion that is both unmistakable and not easily compromised. Any profession that wants to encourage its innovators must address this question: How can the widest range of distinctive styles be tolerated while the excesses of individual style that can destroy goals and objectives are curtailed?

Finally, it is important to recognize that differing styles may not be congenial. An "analytic" can sometimes drive a "gestalt" up the wall, and an "up tight" can give ulcers to someone who "hangs loose" (and vice versa). A profession should recognize the need to accommodate such conflicting types to environments that try to maximize their contributions and minimize their mutually induced traumas. On the other hand, it would be tragic for any profession to be identified with one type to the exclusion of all others; and indeed all sorts of styles can be found among the consumers and providers of service. To avoid unnecessary friction in the delivery of a service, therefore, provision must be made to bring workers and recipients with complementary styles together.

DEGREES OF SKILL

USING THE FOUR dimensions of skill as a framework, we can differentiate among preprofessional (technician), professional (master), and advanced professional (expert) levels of skill. When a worker is expected to operate from fairly well established rules — following directives and commands, adhering to agency style, and utilizing tested techniques and tools of practice — her performance is preprofessional. When she is expected to operate from principles whose justifications are to be found in value-related commendations and theory-based propositions — adhering to professional as well as agency styles and utilizing various methods of intervention — the judgments required are professional. When the worker is expected to consider alternative theoretical formulations and conflicting ethical imperatives — adhering to personal as well as professional and agency styles — and to design a program of action utilizing diverse methods as appropriate, she must demonstrate advanced professional skill. Naturally, any one worker may not only show skill at varying levels in each of the four dimensions but also develop increased skill in each. Our framework, however, focuses upon what is to be done — not upon who does it — in defining levels of skill.

Finally, it should be stressed that skill in professional practice is subject to all the societal and cultural constraints that affect recipient and worker alike. Class, race, sex, and cultural differences necessarily influence one's concept of what is to be valued, what is to be believed, what is to be accepted, and what is to be done. For practical reasons, social workers should be open to a catholic view of skill, lest the profession justifiably be labeled parochial.

»»   ««

As a first approximation, the measurement of skill provides a useful framework for ordering the tools for thought in professional work; but for the worker, so ordering may inhibit a more dynamic appreciation of what practice is all about rather than promoting it. To move the analysis forward to another level, we must consider the mental processes enhanced by these tools. How the worker reasons in practice, how she puts her reasoning to use in arriving at a definition of unmet need, assessing the possible interventions that can be employed in meeting the need, and applying the methods whereby the work is accomplished are complex questions. In Part 3, I discuss each of these facets of the reasoning process in the worker's practice.

»» ««

PART III

Work As Action

CHAPTER TEN

»»   ««

Understanding the Elements of Work

In CHAPTER 1, I considered that working at a profession entails the expenditure of scarce resources, not the least of which is the skill of the practitioner. To warrant such expenditures, a case must be made in favor of altering some existing condition. We noted that the case will be less than persuasive if the following requirements are not met: *(1)* the condition exists and can be described; *(2)* some group in control of resources wishes to improve the condition; *(3)* there is some means to bring about the improvement intended; *(4)* there is willingness to allocate the resources necessary to activate the means so as to achieve the desired end; *(5)* the object of the effort is able and willing, or can be led to participate in the process whereby the change is to be brought about. When the situations described in *(1)* and *(2)* develop, an unmet need is said to exist. When *(3)* and *(4)* are added, a program to provide service is said to exist. Only when *(5)* is present along with the other prerequisites can a service come into being. Consider some of the complicating factors that affect each of these requirements.

THE CONDITION EXISTS
AND CAN BE DESCRIBED

Things are not always what they seem. Not every child sucking his thumb, looking glum, and sitting in a crib reeking of urine is necessarily emotionally and physically deprived. Not every youngster traipsing barefoot along a city street littered with dog droppings, broken glass, pot holes, and cracked sidewalks is in want of shoes. Not every family living in a run-down slum building, with inadequate bathroom facilities and heating is anxious to move. As most of us have noticed, not all conditions we ourselves find deplorable are necessarily so to those most affected by them.

To state that a condition in need of change exists—and to make the statement stick—may require far more study than is needed to describe the obvious. In 1945, for example, I observed the multi-unit housing in the Wurli district of Bombay—buildings without inside toilets, without window panes, without running water, without heat. When I contrasted the residents of these dwellings with the thousands of flimsily dressed, emaciated, disease-ridden persons who dwelt permanently on the streets surrounding these houses, I realized how, in some circumstances, a slum dwelling can be a privileged home.

Evaluations of conditions are as much a function of an anticipated future as of a current state. When we locate a condition in time and place, it may be far more important to mark the direction of its development and the rate at which it is changing than merely to describe the condition itself. Public housing inspectors are responsible for determining if poor housekeeping, with the resulting spread of vermin, foul odors, and destruction of facilities, warrants eviction of the offending family. Evidence suggests that inspectors are less likely to recommend such drastic action if the persons responsible for maintaining the apartment seem to be trying to improve their housekeeping practices than they are when the tenants blame their failure to maintain adequate standards on factors outside their control.[1] The police officer on a neighborhood beat is more likely to book a juvenile for some nuisance violation if the youngster hassles him than he is if the boy shows appropriate contrition.[2] The actual deviant behavior may be unacceptable in either case, but judgments about its reprehensibility will be based on expectations of future behavior.

Omissions in the description may so distort the observation as to make it meaningless or misrepresent it entirely. What can be more reprehensible than a mother leaving her child to die of starvation? In Behar, during the famine of 1943 to 1945, I saw such mothers; but I could only admire their heroism. In some villages, I saw infants clutched tightly to their mothers' breasts, their mouths clamped on the dead nipples of the starved mothers. In Bengal, during this same famine, a group of starving children and adults admonished us when we sought to force desperately needed food into the mouths of some spindly-legged, swollen stomached, youngsters. The most emaciated-looking youngsters were too far gone to be able to swallow. Others who could still swallow selfishly but correctly viewed our efforts as unforgivable waste. An incomplete description of these actual happenings could grossly misrepresent their meaning, even though it remained accurate in detail.

1. Harold Lewis and Mildred Guinessy, *Helping the Poor Housekeeper in Public Housing* (Philadelphia: Friends Neighborhood Guild, 1964).

2. I. Piliavin and S. Briar, "Police Encounters with Juveniles," *American Journal of Sociology* 70 (September 1964): 206–14.

Some deplorable conditions can only be inferred since they are not likely to be directly observable. The absence of food from a refrigerator, the absence of bed-covering and storage space, the infant alone in an apartment — each may show neglect more vividly than some overt measure like truancy, scanty clothing, or malnutrition.[3] The diabetic who needs special foot-care may reveal the extent of her self-care more accurately if she is asked to show the actual utensils she uses to wash her feet than she will if she is asked, "How often do you wash your feet?"[4] These examples suggest the complexities that can make it difficult to achieve supposedly simple descriptions of conditions that are thought to be deplorable.

Many factors, individually or in combination, can influence the judgment of a condition to be altered. For example, a threat to the maintenance of a family may result from changes in health (emotional and physical), economic circumstances, living arrangements, social relationships (community), or family and household composition. Lacks in any of these areas can threaten the structural stability of the family by inhibiting the performance of essential roles by one or more of its members. To judge this condition adequately would entail detailed observation of the factors that contribute to the threat. Otherwise, the other requisites for service to be rendered will not be met.

Let us grant that an adequate and acceptable description of the condition to be altered can be made and that the condition is indeed deplorable. Next, some group in control of resources

3. Harold Lewis, "Identification of Neglect," in "Designing More Effective Protective Services," ed. Harold Lewis, Julius Jahn, and Julia Ann Bishop (Philadelphia: University of Pennsylvania School of Social Work Research Center, 1967), pp. 9–16.

4. Harold Lewis, *The Diabetic Patient* (Providence: Rhode Island Council of Community Services, 1955).

must wish to improve on the condition. Typically, when social services are required, this group will be a social agency.

In theory, it is possible to include this condition (for example, threat to an intact family) on a list of other conditions falling within the range of an agency's purposes. Moreover, it should be possible to designate the various states of each such condition that may be uncovered and the degree of improvement required to make them acceptable. Had we the knowledge to construct such lists, their cross-classification would provide two useful definitions. It would identify both those conditions (or states) in need of improvements and the levels at which agency interventions should normally be initiated. In other words, such a cross-classification would constitute the agency's perception of unmet need. At the other extreme, those states associated with goals or levels that meet community norms for remediation of the condition would define the criteria for termination of service—that is, the point at which a deficiency no longer qualifies as an unmet need. The distance separating the first of these states (for a given condition) from the second would encompass the range of unmet needs for which the agency is willing to expend its resources. The gap between actual goals for termination and ideal goals represents the difference between goals *of* agency work and goals *for* agency work. This gap provides a measure of the extent to which an agency's performance falls short of an agency's promise.

Individuals and social institutions (as well as agencies) arrive at their definitions of unmet needs and their criteria of eligibility and termination in a similar manner. An individual sets restrictions on how a condition must appear to make claims on the work to be done. An entire child welfare system may do likewise. It should be noted that these criteria are the basis for setting standards by which work can be judged, and for evaluating the effectiveness of the work as well.

A GOAL CAN BE SPECIFIED

Decisions that determine whether an unmet need exists are influenced by political, economic, and social restraints affecting individual, organization, and community preferences. The circumstances under which a condition becomes an unmet need can best be understood in the context of the class, cultural, ethnic, sexual, and racial conflicts that permeate all evaluations of need in our society. For this reason, failure to consider the history of the condition, prior efforts to deal with it, and the context in which it is currently evolving, can result in myopic or utopian visions of what is desirable or promote logical blind spots—with a resultant failure to consider reasonable goals. Time and energy are needed to gain the necessary perspective. Most often, both are in short supply.

Goals are rarely attainable through a single program or a combination of short-lived programs. Most often, objectives are set, which the worker hopes to achieve. It is supposed that when all these objectives have in fact been achieved, the goal toward which they are directed will also be achieved. For example, a job-training program may be initiated to increase the skills of its participants and improve their work habits. Although it might be assumed that if both these objectives were achieved the trainees would be eligible for and could find employment (goal), recent experience suggests that often this is not the case.[5] Objectives may be achieved even though the goals are not reached.

5. For example, *Social Services: Do They Help Welfare Recipients Achieve Self-Support or Reduced Dependency?* Report to the Congress by the Comptroller General (Washington, D.C.: Department of Health, Education and Welfare, 1973), pp. 70–78.

Objectives are most likely to be achieved when policies and procedures assure adherence to a practice that has been especially designed for the purpose intended. In turn, tasks assigned and activities engaged in provide evidence that work is being done. The hierarchical structure that relates the work being done to the goal sought is complex; and in practice, it often frustrates pursuit of the goal rather than facilitating it.

The criteria by which one can judge whether a goal has been reached are difficult to identify and still more difficult to measure. What is more, they often fail to gain universal acceptance. For this reason, most accountability procedures at best achieve judgments in relation to objectives; rarely, if ever, do they do so in relation to goals.

Although goals focus attention on purpose, they are justified by reference to values. Because values and their derivatives (ethical imperatives and commendations) are rarely considered crucial to an analysis of goals and objectives, they receive only passing attention — usually when a crisis develops in relation to some violation of ethical behavior. As with the relation of objective to goal, the goal may be realized even when the value that inspired it is not.

RESOURCES AS A MEANS
TO BRING ABOUT
THE IMPROVEMENT INTENDED

Social work as a resource represents a portion of a community's productivity and product intended to meet human welfare needs.[6] In the aggregate, social work

6. Harold Lewis, "The Social Service Commodity in the Inflationary 80's" (Paper presented at Family Service Association of America Workshop for Directors of Professional Services, Toronto, Ontario, 1980).

resources rarely achieve the level of a substantial investment, yet allocations of these resources involve contending community interests in difficult decision-making processes. More often than not, social workers have less to say about how their skill, as a resource, will be used, than do many comparable professions. Since most allocations of this resource are made through the budgets of social agencies (public and private, sectarian and non-sectarian), decisions reflect the preferences of community leaders of various persuasions regarding what social workers should do far more than the workers' own sense of what they can and want to do.

At any one time, identifiable human needs in a community will appear to exceed the resources available to meet them. The demands of contending sectors of the community—each with its own pressing unmet needs—are supposed to be brought into momentary balance by the priority decisions reflected in the allocations made. This is a political process; it may or may not be a rational process.

Agency social work resources, having been provided through this process of allocation, carry with them community expectations shaped by the values and mores of the allocating bodies. These expectations may or may not coincide with those held by the workers and recipients involved in the rendering of services. This variety of expectations necessarily assures limitations on the uses to which social work may be put.

As a means toward an end, resources are combined into programs and incorporate sophisticated methodologies into practice. Skilled work is required to assure not only that targeted groups benefit from the resources expended but also that appropriate methods be used to implement the program. The allocations provided are often insufficient for the programs as they were designed, and those responsible for these programs cannot maintain the quality of work required to achieve the purposes intended.

When they are cross-tabulated, the goals and objectives of

either an agency or an individual, as well as the resources for service available, provide a detailed statement of the program of service. Unequal cell loadings highlight each program's priorities in allocating its resources, and a periodic view of cell distributions shows the direction and degree of change that characterizes the program. Although this matrix can help in an evaluation of the contribution of a social work resource to the purposes of the agency, it is rarely used in this way.

Interesting possibilities for analysis occur when social work resources are related to the conditions to be changed. If one listed the types of intervention judged to be effective in altering its state in the direction of the program's goals for each condition, an assessment typology would result.[7] Moreover, such a listing would define the competence required for practice. The sum of worker competence required to effect change in two or more conditions would suggest needed generic skills, and those unique to certain conditions would suggest specific skills. Implicit in this formulation are causal assumptions providing the rationale for the interventions designated for each condition. The organization of these assumptions into a coherent, logically related whole could suggest the practice science justifying the interventions employed. For the present, neither such a typology nor a coherent practice science has been developed in social work.

These brief analyses of the elements of work are intended as a warning against a too simplistic view of what this work is all about. They may suffice, at this point, to highlight issues relating to the knowledge, value, and practice facets of professional social work skill. Of course, all work involving individual judgments takes on the coloration of different styles; but by design these analyses did not consider the quality of work. For the present, it is enough to consider that style does

7. Max Siporin, *Introduction to Social Work Practice* (New York: Macmillan Co., 1975), pp. 219–50.

help shape the character of the work done—as Chapter 8 sought to demonstrate.

SERVICE

No discussion of the elements of social work is complete without some consideration of the way it brings service into being. Given the prerequisites noted, work can result in a service being rendered when a relationship is established between a potential recipient and the social worker. Through such a relationship, resource and need are brought together; and the relationship is kept intact by the recipient's need for help and the worker's offer of both professional skill and other tangible resources to meet this need. The ensuing exchange (who controls it; whose goals are pursued; who determines its duration and depth; and who chooses the resources to be expended) is hardly simple, containing as it does the essence of what professional competence is all about. Not only the requirements the would-be recipient must meet in order to avail himself of the resources offered but also the requirements the worker must meet in order to make these resources available may strain the relationship and threaten its cohesion. The result of this worker-recipient interaction, which exists in neither of them alone, is service.

To equate service solely with the allocated resources of agency programs is a mistake. Although service incorporates community resources into the worker-recipient relationship, it also provides a major source of the social support needed to develop and sustain that relationship and to instill in it the expectation of a social response to individual need brought to it by the recipient. The provision of a concrete social resource through service carries the potential for meeting need without hindrance and on its own terms. Because it takes the form of a unique and original experience (like all significant relationships), service likewise carries the potential for psychological help; but the extent to which it realizes both these potentials is determined by the appropriateness of the resource to recipient need and the skill with which the two are blended. Service ends when the requirements worker and recipient must both meet ask more than the exchange of resource and need can justify. When this happens, either of the parties (or both) if free to do so will terminate the relationship.

>> <<

Having identified the elements of work that constitute its essentials and noted how these elements combine to generate the definition of need, the assessment of the problem, the intervention to be used, and the program through which service will be rendered, I next consider the mental work entailed in these aspects of a skilled professional practice.

»» ««

CHAPTER ELEVEN

Interventions, Assessment, Outcome, and an Approach to Practice

THE WORKER SEEKS guidance to assure the economic use of her finite resources; but such guidance cannot be given without some prior indication of the scope of the activities that will require her interventions. Whatever program encapsulates these limits (storing perspectives on these limits in memory) is the sum of the intervention procedures formulated to respond to the problem conditions of recipients.[1]

INTERVENTIONS

INTERVENTIONS — actions taken by the worker in response to the recipient's problem condition — include *strategies and tactics*.[2] Intervention strategies link the variety of lesser objectives and lead ultimately to final achievement of the change in the problem condition that made social work services necessary in the first place. A strategy includes an overview of

1. A. N. Soholov, "Studies of the Speech Mechanisms of Thinking," in *Contemporary Soviet Psychology*, ed. Michael Cole and Irving Waltzman (New York: Basic Books, 1969), p. 567.
2. Florence Hollis, *Casework: A Psychosocial Therapy* (New York: Random House, 1964), Chaps. 3, 4; Martin Bloom, *The Paradox of Helping: Introduction to The Philosophy of Scientific Practice* (New York: John Wiley & Sons, 1975), Chap. 10.

the entire engagement of worker and recipient from its beginning to its termination. Intervention tactics concern the variety of tasks completed in the course of the service transaction. Tactics make differential use of techniques; they include work units (or tasks), activity units, and interactions— all dovetailed to the unique requirements of the service process. Strategies and tactics are circumscribed by function, tasks by roles. Tasks are defined by actions unified as sets of activities. Activity units can be measured in individual encounters; and the interactions that make up activities are linked by available modes of performance.

To define an action program in terms of its interventions requires a complex conceptualization. It must analyze the "What am I to do?" and "How am I to do it?" questions for particular classes of service requests. Because such programs are useful only to the extent that their predicted consequences achieve a desired outcome, they draw upon theoretical models that pattern distinctive events into meaningful wholes. They necessarily depend on knowledge of "what" and "what for" to provide relative certainty about which interventions promise to achieve desired changes. For example, a program of action intended to meet a recipient's need for substitute home management in a situation where circumstances prevent the mother from filling essential family functions would include the following: determining eligibility; matching an available homemaker to the family; orienting the family and the homemaker to requirements and limitations in their relationship; sustaining the relationship through counseling services; and arranging for its termination when it is no longer required. In any case, the program particularizes these necessary ingredients and results in a unique pattern that fits the individual situation.[3]

3. Alfred Kadushin, "Assembling Social Work Knowledge," in *Building Social Work Knowledge*, Report of a Conference (New York: National Association of Social Workers, 1964), pp. 16–37.

It is not difficult to imagine the multiplicity of uncertainties a worker must manage in her effort to anticipate the events of a single case. She must act on the basis of knowns whose predictive validity is determined not by 'causal laws' (in the sense that these terms are used in the theoretical sciences) but by statistical probabilities based on relatively large numbers of cases. Expectations that hold for aggregates are often weak in predicting events in individual cases, but they are characteristically the best 'knowns' available to the worker as she develops her program.

Programs that give meaning to priority decisions in a helping process can be viewed as processes in themselves. In their final form, which is the product of the experiences that shape them, they often do not resemble their anticipated form. It is moot whether the program shapes the allocation of resources to the helping process or the experienced process shapes the program. Discussing the concept of truth and its lasting or transitory character with respect to the phenomena with which social workers deal, Herbert Aptekar notes:

> What was "true" at the beginning of a case, from the standpoint of both client and worker, is often no longer true at the middle phase or ending. I refer here not just to the beliefs of both client and worker but to changing external circumstances. Our "truth" will not stand still, so to speak, but changes, even from interview to interview. The parent who hits his child for running in front of a car yesterday may be ashamed of his action today. The "fact" that the child ran in front of the car is incontrovertible and the fact is and remains that the parent hit the child. What we are faced with, however, is the difference between the way the parent felt yesterday and today—it is in a way, an eternally elusive truth—a truth constantly to be sought. No sooner do we have it pinned down than it is no longer 'the truth, the whole truth, and nothing but the truth.' In our case truth seems to be in a constant state of being created and that is what makes it so elusive. I think we must pursue it, but we must be conscious of the fact that it is always a step ahead of us, so to say.[4]

4. Herbert Aptekar, personal communication, February 20, 1970.

There can be little doubt that the reality with which the worker's program of action must be concerned is elusive. A program intended to facilitate and direct interventions in uncertain circumstances should provide for unanticipated consequences. Execution of the program would hardly merit discussion if it entailed only carrying out prescribed tasks in a predetermined sequence of activities, all of which were anticipated in the initial programming of the worker–recipient relationship. In fact, a program that gives meaning to priority choices in professional practice rarely shows this pattern.

A worker does not normally develop her program of action alone. She discusses her intentions with a colleague or a supervisor, and she typically seeks to arrive at both its initial formulation and its subsequent reformulations jointly with the recipient. As her practice puts the program into action, she evaluates its consequences (with the recipient's, and possibly her colleagues', participation) and modifies her activities in the light of experience. In one sense, because it is the product of various interested participants, the worker's program is actually the coordination of different programs. In another, it is the skeleton of a process that is formed only as experience adds flesh to its bones and breathes life into its body. In still another sense, the program is a rational directive for the ordering of possibilities—for the choice of priorities.

A worker must distinguish the action program she helps create for the recipient from the personal plan she makes to give meaning and direction to her inner-directed priority decisions. The personal plan considers the necessary actions dictated by the program. In all probability, the plan and the program will evolve concurrently from the same experiences (and these experiences will include the contingencies each requires for the implementation of the other); but personal plans will primarily reflect the worker's preferences. Her evaluations of her reaction to the recipient and of the demands on her personal resources she anticipates from their relationship will influence her preferences. The worker's doubts and apprehensions about her capacities and her comfort in living with these doubts will also affect her choices. For these reasons, the program for action and the personal plan should be regarded as distinct but related.

Here, too, the worker needs to recover from memory the rules and principles to guide her in developing her personal plan or in choosing from among plans already stored in memory. Even under ideal circumstances, planning is a complex process. Personal plans—linked as they must be to the emotional, intellectual, and social constraints that make up the personality and social attributes of the worker—are possibly still more complex. Such plans draw on the total life experience of the individual worker, not merely her professional circumstance. In relation to her personal plan, the worker's unique attributes, cultural background, and personal involvements appear to serve a crucial orienting function; and practice theory and ethical preferences sharpen the focus of this orientation. The storage and recovery of rules and principles associated with the composition of plans seems to be a difficult and time-consuming process. It is therefore likely that workers often choose among possibilities and establish priorities without meaningful personal plans. "Playing it by ear," "taking chances," "seeing what will happen," "hoping for the best," and a host of other expressions capture the uncertainties that characterize a worker's inner doubts as much as they describe her recognition of unpredictable realities with which she must contend in practice.

In the fullest meaning of the term, self-awareness can assist a worker to appreciate the particular orientation her own personality, culture, and social experience are likely to lend to her choice of personal plans. The suggestions of her supervisor and of her colleagues may increase her ability to weigh possibilities, and practice in which similar demands have been met may also prove useful. In any case, this complex inner-directed process remains shrouded in mystery and badly needs systematic research.

ASSESSMENT

IF INTERVENTION procedures inform and give meaning to priority decisions, assessments are the necessary link between these procedures and desired outcomes of service. An assessment scheme should *(1)* identify the key elements in the problematic situation; *(2)* relate these elements in propositional statements that explain the specific problem conditions to be altered; *(3)* suggest the appropriate intervention procedures and program of action for achieving the desired changes in the problem-conditions; and *(4)* explicitly or implicitly designate the desired consequences of the service. Such a scheme is an ideal not readily achieved in social work practice.

It has been more than a half-century since Mary Richmond sought to provide a scientific basis for social work practice in her classic study, *Social Diagnosis;* and since then much thought and effort have been devoted to the development of diagnostic typologies.[5] At different times, the practice approaches favored by social workers have identified different elements, depending on which underlying theory designated which factor as key to an understanding of the recipient's problematic situation. Each of these approaches has been

5. Samuel Finestone, "Issues Involved in Developing Diagnostic Classifications for Casework," in *Casework Papers*, (New York: Family Service Association of America, 1960), pp. 139–54; Ruth F. Smalley, *Theory for Social Work Practice* (New York: Columbia University Press, 1967), p. 134; Hollis, *Casework*, Chap. 31; Max Siporin, *Introduction to Social Work Practice* (New York: Macmillan Co., 1975), Chap. 9.

proposed and pursued, each has focused on one or more distinctive attributes of recipients and their environment, and each has proposed a distinctive typology to serve as an assessment tool.[6] Given the complexity of the phenomena with which the worker must contend and the varieties of programs in which social work skills are utilized, however, it is not surprising that no single approach has provided a unifying theoretical foundation for a satisfactory assessment scheme applicable to the full range of social work practice.

Social workers may agree with Ruth Smalley's statement:

> That diagnosis, or understanding of the phenomenon served, is most effective for all the social work processes which is related to the use of the service; which is developed, in part, in the course of giving the service with the engagement and participation of the clientele served; which is recognized as being subject to continuous modification as the phenomenon changes; and which is put out by the worker for the clientele to use, as appropriate, in the course of the service.[7]

Opinions will nevertheless differ about what constitutes an "understanding of the phenomenon served"; that is, what is a sound and effective assessment. Whereas this question cannot be answered without considerable knowledge of and

6. For example, Robert W. Roberts and Robert H. Nee, eds., *Theories of Social Casework* (Chicago: University of Chicago Press, 1970); Catherine B. Papell and Beulah Rothman, "Social Group Work Models: Possession and Heritage," *Journal of Education for Social Work* 2 (1966): 66–78; for a summary discussion, see Siporin, *Social Work Practice*, pp. 136–56; for a view focusing on special areas of social work practice, see *Social Work* 26, no. 1 (January 1981), second special issue on conceptual frameworks.

7. Smalley, *Theory for Social Work Practice*, p. 134; for a detailed application of an assessment framework congenial with Smalley's discussion, see Sr. Mary Paul Janchill, *Guidelines to Decision-Making in Child Welfare* (New York: Human Services Workshop, 1981), pp. 7–34.

agreement about goals and objectives, such knowledge appears to be unevenly developed with respect to the different programs, problems, and processes that make claims on skills of social workers.

However one arrives at an assessment and however one employs it in practice, no approach to practice can make light of the effort entailed in assembling the variety of facts and feelings that go into defining a recipient's situation. The assessment statement serves only as an intellectual aid, something to organize complex data into compositions that store definitions of the recipient's situation. Through association with analogs in memory, such compositions also facilitate the recovery of rules and principles for the selection and application of interventive procedures. A professional practice that lacks assessment typologies leaves the practitioner confronting an almost insurmountable task—she must continuously master these complex materials and form them into compositions, a requirement that can quickly exhaust her intellectual and emotional energies. For this reason, those approaches to practice that have taken hold and gained support among practitioners usually offer a conceptual terminology full of nominal categories to serve diagnostic ends.

In a practice totally subsumed by rule-governed commands, an assessment typology may demonstrate exact correspondence with associated intervention procedures. This is especially so when assessment requires categorization to orient the worker to the general attributes that characterize the service engagement and where standard procedures are intended to deal with these attributes. Many routine operations in rendering social services illustrate this pattern. Typically, these operations become repetitive and call for limited judgment on the part of the worker. When a service request calls for substantial individual judgment and demands more skilled practice, a worker who fails to pursue the variations that distinguish this request from others within the same category appears to be using typology as a crutch rather than a tool. By facilitating the storage and recovery process, a sound assessment scheme should free the worker to consider more carefully the unique aspects of individual requests and to tailor the process of intervention to fit the peculiarities of each instance of a class of cases.

OUTCOMES

THE INADEQUACIES of assessment schemes and intervention procedures in social work practice have been major stumbling blocks to the further development of professional competence. In part, these limitations are attributable to a lack of knowledge about problems confronted in practice and possible modes of intervention. In part, these limitations also stem from confusion about the goals to be sought and about the outcome measures that can serve as criteria for judging achievement.

Objective measures of consequences are essential before one can make rational choices among alternative modes of action. After making a careful study and analysis of the recipient's circumstances, earlier experiences, expectations, and potential, the worker hopefully uses her knowledge, experience, intuition, and judgment to predict to herself the probable momentum and development of her recipient's behavior and attitudes. Her prediction often changes as service is provided; and it may take the form of a series of short-term expectations that contribute to the formulation of a single long-term expectation. The inner-directed predictions of the worker need neither imply a deterministic view of recipient behavior or of the social context nor assume a rigid, noncreative, restricted view of the potential for change in the service encounter. It does ask of the worker, however, a degree of understanding of the service situation, the presenting problem, and the available means for dealing with the problem that permits an estimate of probable consequences but does not exclude other unanticipated outcomes.

Commendable outcomes that cannot be directly and clearly attributed to a worker's activities hardly offer evidence to support assessment schemes or intervention procedures. Demonstrating a causal relationship between worker-directed activities and changes achieved, however, is quite difficult.[8] For this reason, predictive accuracy—because it provides some basis upon which to assume a causal sequence of means and ends—may be treated as a source of evidence for selecting preferred assessment schemes and intervention procedures. We can assume that when anticipated and desired outcomes are realized according to an a priori rationale, a worker is encouraged to trust the activities associated with these results and therefore wants to experiment further with the tools and procedures that informed these activities. She will have to satisfy herself that the results move in the direction of the goals she hopes to achieve; but the choice of goals—essential to any such logical process for delineating professional preferences—is governed by value considerations, not merely those of fact.

It is sometimes argued that the goals of social work are best stated in terms of justice rather than charity. The efforts of social workers, whatever their modes of practice, are intended to increase recipient opportunities for choice and recipient access to resources commensurate with the need to be met— if equitable opportunity for choice is to be realized. In this

8. During the 1970s, this difficulty was amply documented and reviewed in the literature. An early note of warning was sounded in Elizabeth Herzog, *Some Guidelines for Evaluative Research: Assessing Psycho-Social Change in Individuals* (Washington, D.C.: Department of Health, Education and Welfare, Social Service Administration, Children's Bureau, 1959), pp. 62–71; for a brief discussion, see Gerald Landsberg, William D. Heigher, Roni J. Hammer, Charles Windle, and J. Richard Woy, *Evaluation in Practice* (Rockville, Maryland: National Institute of Mental Health, 1979), pp. 117, 121.

view, the social worker herself is a special type of resource—the recipient's counselor, advocate, and enabler, who seeks always to maximize her client's opportunities to act on his own behalf within a scheme guided by principles of distributive justice. Given distributive justice as a goal, the consequences that would serve as measures of service achievement would only indirectly be evident in cures, in solutions of problems, in satisfactions, or in social and emotional independence. The desired outcome would instead be directly measured by the degree of equity discernable in opportunity achieved—given the constraints of persons and situations over which the recipient (even with the aide of agency resources) has no effective control. In this view, social workers primarily promote the achievement of distributive justice for the recipients of their services, using their skills and agency resources toward this end.

Social work is also perceived as a professional mode of social treatment, functioning in both social institutions and individual practice to assist in the amelioration, elimination, or prevention of personal and social problems. In this view, the goal of service is to help the recipient achieve maximum health and social well-being by supporting, supplementing, and otherwise providing help in personal and social functioning. Assuming responsibility neither for the recipient's self-direction nor for the basic social, economic, and political institutions of the society in which the recipient must cope, the social worker tries to influence and relate the two in a manner that increases the potential of both to advance individual and societal purposes. These views of the goals of social work (like many similar views) are sufficiently abstract in formulation, broad in scope, and ethical in commendation to warrant widespread support among professionals. Unfortunately, such general statements about goals offer little guidance to the worker who is trying to arrive at quantifiable criteria to use as outcome measures in daily practice.

It is possible, however, to reduce these general intentions

to measurable objectives, which can be taken as concrete manifestations of the outcomes that should follow if these goals were in fact realized. Some variables that might achieve a useful level of specificity for child welfare, for example, are the following. The lower the numerical value of the variable, the more favorable the client's situation.

1. The number of days during which a person under 21 years of age has been removed from the custody of living parents by action of Juvenile or Family Court.
2. The number of days that any adult is confined in a custodial institution because of conviction on charges of abuse of a child.
3. The number of days that a person under 21 years of age spends in a hospital as a result of injuries for which according to the medical records an adult is responsible.
4. The number of days that a child of school age is absent from school; or is attending a school or class in which he has been placed for reason of educational retardation or disciplinary problems.
5. The number of days of residence in a public or private institution for the care and treatment of a psychiatrially classified mental illness or disability.
6. The number of days a person is confined to bed, hospital, or other institution due to any illness or disability other than (3) or (5).
7. The number of days a person is confined to jail or other correctional institution, other than (2).
8. The amount that a person's income, or the per capita income of members of a household, is less than the per capita income of all persons of the same age group and sex in the community, etc.

If the worker finds these criteria too broad for her purposes, she can make them more specific by seeking evidence to assure her that one can identify changes which improve the recipient's condition as a consequence of her efforts. These criteria might include the following:

1. Housing arrangement, including heat, refrigeration, laundry facilities, security from intruders, housekeeping, shopping, repair and maintenance.
2. Eating routines, including location, regularity, dietary balance, preparation.
3. Sleeping accommodations, including own bed, quilt, adequate cover.
4. Work history, including its nature, stability, satisfaction, adequacy of income.
5. Other income sources.
6. Physical health (injuries, routine medical care, medications) and necessary appliances (glasses, dentures).
7. Adjustment (including symptoms of emotional stress, personal care, decision making, planning, appearance, outlook), and interpersonal relationships, (including friends, social and recreational activities, visits and help with friends and relatives), organization of time.[9]

From an agency's point of view, if the latter evidences of change are shown to be highly associated with or directly contributory to the former, they may result in broader criterion measures that the community is likely to accept as justification for continued support of its services; and a fairly rational and feasible definition of *goals* will be achieved. In some important ways, such a formulation would meet the require-

9. Ben Ami Gelin and Julius A. Jahn, "Research Design," in "Designing More Effective Protective Services: Appendix," ed. Harold Lewis, Julius Jahn, Shankar Jalaija, and Ben Ami Gelin (Philadelphia: University of Pennsylvania School of Social Work Research Center, 1967), pp. 4–5; see also Janchill, *Guidelines to Decision-Making*, pp. 37–91.

ments we earlier identified as necessary if assessment and interventive typologies useful for practice are to be achieved.

The methodological complexity of any procedure that seeks to identify and measure criterion variables and associate them with the intervention procedures intended to promote their achievement need not be pursued here. Of interest for this discussion, however, is the inquiry the worker puts to herself about her personal goals in this activity. How does she arrive at what she will seek to achieve, and what does she accept as evidence that her efforts are appropriate and that they lead in the direction she intends?

WORKER GOALS

A SOCIAL WORKER is normally aware of the range of problems that complicate the lives of normal, relatively untroubled human beings. She owes this awareness to her educational preparation, to her professional practice, and most important, to her own experience. Without having to discover it for herself in each new service relationship, she knows that she cannot hope to eliminate a recipient's problems in living. At best, she can help him deal with those problems for which her services may be appropriate. Sometimes, all the worker's professional skill seems to be focused on restating a problem in a form that is more manageable for the recipient, given his capacity and motivation for coping with problems. The recipient's choice of agency, program, or service in effect serves as a screening mechanism and reduces the scope of what must be attended to in deciding just which service may make a legitimate claim on the agency's and the worker's resources. Granted all the procedures and requirements that further limit what the recipient can realistically expect, the worker must ask herself, "What outcomes are possible for this recipient? Which of them would this recipient be motivated to seek? Which can the worker hope to promote? Which can the agency accept as evidence of its program intention? Which can the community feel justified in supporting?"

She will decide on her inner-focused set of criterion variables by questioning herself. This process is integral to the formulation by which she has already stored compositions arranged in response to these questions: "What am I to do now? How am I to do it? In what order ought I do what I can do in this situation?" The stored analogs that clue her to what she is to do operate by associating alternatives with probable outcomes, usually of a short-run nature. Thus, if the recipient's inquiry suggests a request for child placement, the recovered rule will first suggest the completion of an application in anticipation that the short-term outcome will consist of initiating the service relationship and second clue the worker to a possible assessment of how she is to proceed. The "How am I to do it?" self-inquiry attaches the composition to its analog, recovering associated intervention rules that provide short-term responses congenial to the stage of diagnostic insight thus far achieved. The third question—the priority question—poses strategic choices to be recovered and probably suggests only partial approximations of long-term outcomes to be sought. These choices will nevertheless introduce compositions that tap related strategic goals into the worker's inner awareness—goals previously derived from the unraveling of similar strategies. At this point, the worker's plan of service takes shape.

This description of a worker's thinking postulates an inner-directed inquiry process whereby a worker gets in touch with her personal criterion variables. Because it is only a hypothesis unsupported by empirical evidence, we should use caution in assigning to it any significance, except that it might be used as a heuristic model of the process, which to my knowledge has not been studied in professional literature. Such an exercise in imagination, however, can be justified by the need to distinguish between the objective measures of outcome so crucial to evaluative research and the inner-selected criteria necessary as evidence of the worker's "success" when she is queried about the efficacy of her efforts.

When a worker is asked to describe cases in which she has been successful, she will often provide an assessment of both the condition she sought to affect and the interventions that worked, giving selected examples of the behavior and attitude of the recipient and a before-and-after contrast that suggests a causal sequence with measurable and desirable results. Pressed further, she may also point out how the results she achieved could be extrapolated to show how broader community goals of service would probably result from the actual service rendered.

On the other hand, when the worker is asked to describe cases in which she has been unsuccessful, she will often present her assessment of the condition to be affected in such a way as to anticipate its irremedial characteristics and pay almost scant attention to the limitations of intervention procedures. She is also likely to suggest that recipient attitude and behavior led to inappropriate request for service or imply some serious limitation to recipient motivation or capacity that in turn made an offer to help irrelevant or pointless.

In the former instance, the worker uses self-selected outcome variables to judge her work and find it satisfactory. In the latter, she focuses on objective criterion measures for she is not equipped to answer the trio of self-directed questions previously noted; therefore she directs her evaluation outward and states it in terms of the recipient's problems and circumstances that frustrated any effort at help. It thus appears that when the worker judges success, she sees it in terms of what she *believes* works for her; and when she judges failure, she sees it in terms of what she *knows* does not work for the recipient.

Although these perspectives complement each other, they leave unanswered essential questions about a logical procedure both for determining criterion measures and for relating them to interventive procedures. At a minimum, what does *not* work for the worker (in terms of her skills and resources) and what *does* work for the recipient, (in terms of his strengths and circumstances) must be included in explanations of results achieved. Further, whatever explanations of outcomes are found necessary and sufficient, they should satisfy the community's expectations about goals of services if they are to sustain a valid claim on husbanded resources for which other competing allocation requests are always present.

In her orientation to the values of the profession and the agency, and in her own personal values, a social worker stores for recovery the norms of the community that purchases her services and judges their effects. Inevitably, however much the worker may personally deviate from these norms — or reject them or find them inappropriate to her recipient's circumstances — the definition of 'need' justifying a request for service implies that the recipient's condition carries some valuation based on existing community norms. Thus, as the worker defines the recipient's problem, she composes for storage a perspective that associates the recipient's condition with an analog of acceptable goal-valuations already present in memory and recovered along with appropriate rules and principles for action. It is rare for a worker to need to seek a totally new set of criterion variables in theory and values against which to measure her own views of preferred outcomes.

The different perspectives on valuation that result from the divergence between the relationship of worker and recipient inherent in efforts to 'treat' and the relationship in attempts to assure 'justice,' create a dilemma for the worker. Treatment and cure are intended to identify and solve problems; they orient the worker to measure her success on the basis of her intervention procedures and diagnostic categories — within realistic limits set by a recipient's capacity and motivation. On the other hand, distributive justice implies a three-way relationship in which the worker maintains sufficient distance from both the recipient and the community-agency to maximize opportunity for both to achieve an equity that will benefit both. The latter circumstance is not unlike the adversary procedure in law, in that the worker may feel that her efforts were successful even when the recipient's claims for access are not realized if she has made the best possible presentation of the recipient's claim. Maintaining a certain psychological distance from the recipient may be essential to avoiding a judgment of the recipient rather than his claim and its justifications.

Social work practice nevertheless encourages a worker to seek closeness with the recipient necessary so she can maximize whatever psychological help she can offer. Even so, she must nevertheless maintain the kind of distance that allows her to represent a just claim without prejudicing it because of extraneous factors in the recipient's situation. If justice does not prevail in access to resource and distribution of resource, and in the reward of benefits based primarily on need, it is inevitable that a social worker can fulfill her professional commitment only if she attempts to play both roles in relation to the recipient; but a requirement to do so may be neither emotionally, psychologically, or behaviorally feasible.

Different role requirements are involved in a practice that stresses treatment and cure on the one hand and seeks justice on the other. Nevertheless, the worker must find ways and means to reconcile these roles in pursuing justice and treatment in every phase of her practice. It is difficult to conceive of a principled, helping process involving human relationships that can avoid having to deal with both requirements.

This analysis of intervention, assessment, and outcome suggests convenient, efficient, and useful units for mental storage and recovery of social work knowledge and values. It also requires a means whereby the worker may encapsulate various roles in a framework that facilitates the effective organization of practice principles. One approach to practice that attempts to meet this requirement is based on the view that a variety of roles are subsumed under the umbrella concept of function, from which such roles derive their justification. To illustrate how one integrated practice model has been formulated, the concept of function and its informing principles of practice is futher explored in rounding out this discussion of action. This approach, called the *functional school,* was developed during the late 1930s and early 1940s. Since then, many of its elements have been integrated into other, more current formulations.

THE FUNCTIONAL APPROACH

THE FUNCTIONAL APPROACH is primarily intended to solve a problem central to social work practice: How can one provide the community-sponsored services of social agencies in a manner that assures the opportunity for their maximum utilization by the recipients of services?[10] In common with other social professions, social work has developed under organizational sanction and traditionally depended on organizational resources. It is not surprising therefore that a major approach to professional practice has been concerned with one crucial aspect of organizational effectiveness—the direct rendering of an agency's service to its clientele. Thus the manner in which the problem was stated sets the limits within which the functional approach attempted its solution.

10. For the original article on which this discussion is based, see Harold Lewis, "The Functional Approach to Social Work Practice: A Restatement of Assumptions and Principles," *Journal of Social Work Process* 15 (1966): 115–33. The article contains bibliographic references to key discussions of this approach in the writings of its major advocates.

The Agency

Social agencies can be viewed as institutional expressions of a community's concern for its collective well-being. Although this assumption is not without precedent, for the functional approach it is the essential frame of reference used to define the task of professional social work. The unique role assigned to social work by the community and played by the profession for the community is commonly performed within the context of these institutional forms. Agencies come into being as a result of conscious decisions to allocate a part of the community's resources from public and private sources to meet the welfare needs of its citizens. Once these resources assume the form of evident services supplied by social agencies and their programs, the problem central to the functional approach is posed.

The social agency constitutes the 'given,' the dynamic field of action within which the functional approach expects social work activity to occur. Guiding principles for functional practice will always be framed within this context.

>» «<

The principal participants in the social work activity taking place within this context are the recipient and the social worker.

The Recipient

The recipient's welfare is central to all social work activity. His condition and the need it is judged to reflect provide the basis for community concern and the justification for allocating community resources. The functional approach also assumes that in the final analysis the direction of the recipient's life is dependent upon his own conscious choices and activities. It further assumes that the recipient has an unforseeable potential to solve his own problems although he may need help in realizing this potential. The recipient is viewed within the context of those elements of his situation that can aid him or hinder him in dealing with his problems—in the light of his own history and background, his variety of group associations, and his community role, as citizen. Whereas a specific agency service may be intended to meet the needs resulting from a specific condition (individual or social), if its service is to help the recipient to the fullest, the way in which it is rendered must engage the whole person and include both knowledge and understanding of his situation on the part of the worker. This situation always includes his experience of contact with the worker, and the impact of the "realities" of the agency on him.

The functional approach regarded the recipient as an individual capable of choice and able—no matter how limiting his circumstances or endowment—to exercise that choice. The concept of choice exceeds the narrow sense of selection among predetermined alternatives to include freedom to find in each new helping relationship a range of alternatives—appropriate to the "readiness" of the recipient and maximizing his use of himself as a choosing person. It also includes the need to provide conditions and resources that make choice realizable.

The Worker

In her capacity as staff member of a social agency, a social worker is an agent of whatever part of the community has sanctioned and provided the resource. She is instrumental in making resources available in their 'agency service' form; and she is expected to provide a psychological climate that can initiate and sustain the relationship with the recipient through which service is transacted. It is expected that the relationship that develops in this climate—humanly caring, respectful, and expectant—will maximize the recipient's opportunity for choice and motivate him to use the service to the best of his ability. The worker is also called upon to carry the serious responsibility of feeding back to both agency and community the new understanding of unmet needs and ways of meeting them, generated by each offering of service.

The functional approach assumes that a social worker must seek to affect the way each recipient deals with each problem as he tries to use the agency's service. This assumption directs the worker to encourage the recipient to deal with the conditions that caused him to apply for service in such a way that he increases his capacity for dealing with similar conditions, should they arise in the future. As a professional, the worker should bring to each contact with her recipient not only her knowledge but also the ethical standards of behavior and accepted values and norms of the profession. As citizen, the worker supposedly shares the same obligations and rights with other community members, but she has greater than average capacity (and consequent responsibility) for informed participation in shaping and affecting community social welfare policy.

The Helping Process

Because of its known purpose, the activity of the social worker and the recipient was assumed also to have a necessary coherence and direction. The terms *beginning, middle,* and *ending* served to delineate chronological phases, each with its distinctive significance, in the process elaborated by their interaction. While the agency provided both the setting and the specific focus of social work practice, the recipient–worker interaction generated the process through which the content of practice came alive in time phases.

In addition, the functional approach also assumed that the helping process was further identified by growth potential. Here, the relationship between worker and recipient was the simplest irreducible unit for carrying this potential.

According to the functional approach, growth is generative — a process that makes the recipient aware of and able to use conscious choice rather than a release that permits him to follow some predetermined path. The functional approach assumed that change is inner-directed. Unlike a model that attributes the primary impulse for change to an external source, functional formulations assumed that some inner purpose and impulse on the part of the recipient constantly suggested the direction and change sought by both worker and recipient. The social worker tried to release this inherent potential rather than initiate 'change' and such release was achieved by the joint efforts of the recipient and the social worker. The skill of the social worker thus lay in her ability consciously to establish a professional relationship moving in time that would release the potential of the recipient for dealing more effectively with his own life.

Service

In functional social work, service was a melding of agency, worker, recipient, profession, and community purpose. As a social resource, service carries the potential for "real" help ("realistic meeting of need without hindrance and on its own terms"). Service as a unique and individual experience in relationship — an expression of the way in which resource is provided — carries the potential for psychological help. The extent to which service realized both these potentials was determined both by the appropriateness of resource to need and by the skill with which they were blended in the social work process.

Relating the Elements of the Functional Approach

Thus far, we have identified *(1)* the setting (agency), *(2)* the participants (recipient, worker), and *(3)* service, as elements in the social process encompassed by the functional approach. How are these elements related to one other as they materialize in practice?

In its simplest form, the functional approach visualized a human relationship involving a *social worker as helper,* instrumental to the rendering of an *agency's service* intended to meet a *recipient's need* through a process that maximizes the recipient's opportunity to use the service effectively. These focal concepts were interrelated in a form that permitted their dynamic interdependence to be seen, even though it was not entirely understood. One natural advantage of such a practice-oriented concept is that it can be used to suggest guides for action that permit considerable freedom for original expression but can be adapted to a variety of circumstances while avoiding the implication that they are necessarily based only on what is "known." What is *felt* to be *understood* by the participants can and does serve as an experiential base for consensus on guides for action—or principles. *Acting* on the basis of limited certainties and in relation to newly generated and unforeseen data, was characteristic of the functional approach to practice.

Principles

Principles of functional practice are derived directly from the relationship of elements in the functional approach. Statements about the nature of man, the human condition, the social milieu, institutional organization and structure, needs, resources, and service abound in social work literature generally, and in functional writings as well. The 'knowns' about each of these subjects constitute a substantial body of knowledge that is constantly undergoing reformulation in the behavioral and biological sciences and in the service professions. Functional principles were concerned with the *use* of this necessary knowledge to provide social agency services in a helpful way; and through the process of providing such help, functional social work hoped to make its distinctive contribution to knowledge. Functional principles offered the social worker guides to professional action in her role as participant in the agency-based and recipient-centered drama.

From the many sources providing knowledge for use in practice, social workers receive cues for action which they incorporate into their efforts to provide help. The principles discussed here represent only the essential generalizations of the functional approach. The skill of the functional worker was judged in relation to the appropriate and creative application of these principles in practice. Starting with the assumptions of the functional approach, that social work helping occurs under the auspices of a social agency and that the agency provides the relatively stable 'given' in each helping relationship through which its services are rendered, certain constraints can be noted about the essential requirements agencies must meet to facilitate the helping process:

1. The agency must make clear through its structure, policy, and procedures the kinds of service it offers and the prerequisites for such service, which must be accepted or rejected by the applicant, whether he comes to the agency voluntarily or through the community's concern or requirement.
2. The need the agency is prepared to meet must permit more than one possibility of fulfillment, so that the recipient may choose to meet or not to meet the agency's conditions.
3. The agency carries authority of different kinds and degrees—the recipient's choice is the option on how to use it. For this reason, choices that are held to be expectations of the recipients wishing to use an agency's service require that the agency provide conditions that make such choices possible.
4. The agency must provide the channels and means to

assure continuous review of its purpose, function, policies, structure, procedures, and services. Awareness of and participation in changes in the community's attitudes, resources, and needs—and in its own program and clientele—should provide the basis for the agency's own alteration of goals, standards, methods, and services.

5. The agency must take the responsibility for sharing with the community the accumulated evidence of unmet human need resulting from its efforts on behalf of recipients—standing strongly for the use of such evidence to stimulate new resources and to realign old ones to meet these human needs.

Similarly, the recipient is expected to include in his person and situation certain 'givens,' if the helping process is to eventuate in service rendered. At some point in the process,

1. The recipient must want the help offered through the particular service.
2. The recipient must be able to exercise choice in relation to whether or not he wants to meet the conditions of service required by the agency.
3. The recipient must be able and free to choose his own goals in relation to which he seeks to utilize agency service.

Within the limitations set by these expectations on the part of both agency and recipient, principles of function and process are intended to guide the worker's practice.

Practice

In practice, the principles of process are meaningful as guides to worker performance only when they are consistently related to the particular function of the agency. They include not only the policies, procedures, and conditions of service but also the underlying psychological meaning of that function for both recipient and community in relation to the problems that the service is designed to solve. Similarly, the principles must be seen as governing the interaction of the worker and recipient through a process that continues and develops as it moves toward some kind of closure or culmination. It is assumed that a body of knowledge related to any particular function must be known and used. In the final analysis, what is helpful resides in the interpenetration of function and process carried out by the human medium.

Function

An agency's function must have both range and depth, but the agency, with its clearly defined function and operational policies, must also provide the limits, orientation, and focus necessary for creative performance on the part of both social worker and recipient. It is expected that the recipient will test the limitations inherent in the agency's functions and policies, in order to accept, reject, attempt to control, or modify, trying ultimately to find what he can use of the agency's service and how he can use himself in relation to it. The worker's responsibility as an 'agent' of the agency carrying out its function determines roles she will play in the helping relationship.

Here are three principles:

1. The worker must present what the agency has to offer for the recipient's need as the recipient states this need or is helped to perceive it.
2. The worker must explain the conditions or expectations the recipient must meet in order to avail himself of the agency's resources.
3. The worker must understand the emotions stirred by the

specific function (related to her particular need) — a factor in the living reality between recipient and worker.

In practice, these principles will involve both worker and recipient in an effort to discover whether the problem, as the recipient sees and faces it at the moment, and the agency help the worker is able to give fit together. As alternative resources are considered, the recipient may work out unexpected solutions to his problem. The terms on which help must be given, including the consequences these terms entail for the recipient, will be weighed by both.

Process

Process implies a sequence that orders time. To the extent that time is the medium of the helping process, the aim of the worker is to provide a unique experience in relationship in which time is heightened by limits deliberately utilized. On the assumption that the recipient has his own innate power to change and to use experience selectively to his own ends, one goal of the process is to assure him the opportunity to utilize his own experience in arriving at his own conclusions within the time available to him. The premise that everyone resists the very help he seeks unless he participates in its control permits the recipient to overcome his initial fear of and resistance to any help that affects the self — in brief, it allows time for the psychological dynamics to traverse their natural path and avoids attempting to induce direct change in the recipient, which might serve only to increase his resistance or result in his capitulation to an outer force.

Eleven further principles help to initiate and control this process:

4. The worker must build on the recipient's strengths to face whatever realities are decisive in determining his

own use both of himself and of available resources in relation to the problem he faces upon which he wants to work.

5. The worker must assure the recipient the opportunity to choose his own goal and help him to find that goal rather than act out of fear, guilt, or some other extraneous emotion.

6. The skill of the worker must be focused on the helping process itself, not on discovery or recapitulation of past experience — without denial of the significance of the past, but rather with its inclusion as a relevant factor in understanding the recipient's movement in the present.

7. The worker must continue to focus clearly on the reality of her current relationship with the recipient by helping him face the demands of the present.

8. The worker must personally interject something new to the situation to offer the recipient a new view of it or a new grip on it or a view of himself in it.

9. The worker must offer through and within the helping relationship a new experience for the recipient, in which and around which old patterns of thought, feeling, and behavior — inadequate to the existing need — can be discarded sufficiently to afford a new start toward some personal and social reorganization.

10. The worker must find out what has happened to the recipient as a result of contact with the agency — past or present — to utilize this knowledge for the recipient's movement.

11. The worker must establish sufficient separateness from the recipient so that neither confuses the other with his or her own self. The worker's identification with her agency's function and her acceptance of the role derived from it help her to establish and maintain the necessary separation.

12. The worker must recognize the recipient's right to his

own feelings as indexes of his own values. She must also recognize *her* own feelings as they are generated by the worker–recipient relationship and provide for their effect as the relationship develops.

13. As she expresses her feelings, a worker must concentrate upon the recipient's need to know and experience genuine emotion from another person. Within the relationship, the worker can help the recipient experience and affirm his own feelings and take responsibility for them as he plans and acts on his plans.

Each of these principles is applied to each individual recipient or recipient group through interaction with the worker. When the clientele is a group or when interaction occurs within a group, an additional principle must be noted:

14. The worker's relation to each member is important, but she must modify the many diverse and individual strands of her interaction with the group members so that she has a connection with the group as a whole and enhances members' relationships with each other.

In the functional approach, the psychological dynamics that accompany a recipient's encounter with the appropriate application of these principles by a worker were worked out most clearly in the practice of social casework. Such an application first involved the recipient in acknowledging his need for help, later by unburdening himself in projection, and gradually by taking back into himself (with new tolerance and responsibility) the parts that had been deposited upon others. From the process evolving out of the relationship engendered by the application of these principles, it was expected that the casework recipient in need would shift his relationship to the object that satisfied the need, modify his ways of seeking and controlling it, and find a new relation both to external resources and to his own strength and weakness.

This summary suggests the 'use' orientation that guided the formulations of this approach—intended as it was to bring about some form of social change. Each of the central elements (social agency, worker, resource, need, and recipient use of self) was viewed as an independent condition with predictive potency in relation to the outcome sought. Each was also viewed as tractable through some form of control, approachable within the value base of the social work profession. Each could be assigned relative weights indicative of some value measure. Potentially, the extent of the impact that resulted from the differential application of each element could be gauged. Finally, the approach expected unanticipated consequences primarily involving the object of change.

As a guide for practice, the functional approach left open the range of roles open to the worker—helper, enabler, advocate, mediator, counselor, among others—in fulfilling the purpose of the agency. It provided far less guidance for the private practitioner. Although it offered a well-integrated and systematic rationale, this approach by no means encompassed everything that falls within the substantive intent and methodological concerns of social work.[11]

For example, consider how this approach would define the function and roles of the worker in relation to social action. Over many decades, one heatedly debated issue has been the nature of the relationship between cause and function. Understandably, this issue was of central concern to function-

11. Alvin Gouldner, "Theoretical Requirements of the Applied Social Sciences," in *The Planning of Change*, ed. Warren G. Bennis, Kenneth D. Benne, and Robert Chin (New York: Holt, Rinehart and Winston, 1961), pp. 83–95. This case example of an approach to practice was selected because it offers a well-integrated and systematic rationale that is no longer undergoing significant changes.

alists, and it led to differences in views that persist to this day. The manner in which the issue is raised often reveals the viewpoint of the person raising it. Wondering where the one-to-one helping process stands in the midst of a wave of mass programs and resources in areas that did not exist earlier (i.e., after the influx of new programs associated with the Fair Deal and later with the War on Poverty), a leading advocate of the functional approach asked, "Have we lived through a period of making resources available and may there now be a return to interest in how the individual himself uses these resources, makes them available to himself?"[12] This very question reveals a questioner who assumes that social programs (i.e., making resources available) and personal utilization of these resources occur in a linear or cyclical pattern. From a practice perspective, the role of advocate might be more appropriate to periods when attempts to make more resources available are most important, and the roles of helper and enabler to the periods that follow, when the function calls for greater stress on personal utilization of these resources. The functional approach provided no generalized principles by which to judge which of these periods characterizes a situation in particular areas of human need, in different locations, and with different populations. In the absence of such principles, the practitioner must seek guidance from theory and ethics. If she can find no clarity at that level, she must look to knowledge and values to develop her own program for action in her work.

>»   ««

We have now completed an introduction to the intellec-

12. See Harold Lewis, "The Cause in Function." *Journal of the Otto Rank Association* 2, no. 2 (Winter 1976–77): 17–25.

tual tasks involved in the practice of social work. From the initial discussion of the elements of work, the worker, and the intellectual tools useful in her work, we developed a structure for conceptualizing skill in practice. We then considered in greater depth the difficult intellectual tasks entailed in the application of skill—concluding with one example of approach to practice that sought to incorporate much of what we identified as essential to such a conceptualization.

Undergirding all these discussions are common mental processes that we generally call reasoning. In Chapter 12, I address these reasoning processes, helping to clarify how they enter into the intellectual work involved.

CHAPTER TWELVE

»»   ««

Reasoning in Practice

UNDERPINNING THE WORK DONE and the skill evident in its performance is the worker's capacity for reasoned thought.[1] Intellectual work asks a worker to think clearly and productively so that her efforts further her purposes. Thus far, however, I have deliberately avoided a more detailed analysis of the reasoning process itself, which must now be considered. It seemed sensible to present the structure and tools used in the mental work of the profession before describing, even briefly, the processes that breathe intellectual life into this work.

In a professional practice, most of the important action occurs in the mind of the worker. This observation is not intended to belittle the importance of emotions, talk, physical contact, and manipulation; but it implies that these activities can be understood as manifestations of professional work only to the degree that the reasoning of the practitioner responsible for orchestrating their occurrence is appreciated.[2] In the absence of a need to make judgments, rule-governed behavior dominates, and little professional competence is

1. See Harold Lewis, "Reasoning in Practice," *Smith College Studies in Social Work* 46, no. 1 (1975): 3–15, for the original article on which this discussion is based.

2. Charlotte G. Babcock, "Social Work as Work," *Social Casework* 34, no. (1953): 415–22.

required. Where choices must be made and such choices require informed and purposeful judgments, professional competence is needed. It is appropriate, for this reason, to begin with the mental processes of professional action, review them as the most important part of the action, explicate their characteristics, and observe how they enter into the judgments of the worker.

ASSUMPTIONS

IN ORDER TO practice effectively, the worker must relate herself to what is true rather than to what she wishes to be true. It is also essential to the performance of tasks that realistic appraisal provide the basis for action. In practice, the worker does not discount self-imposed and socially sanctioned distortions; she appreciates them as aspects of her view of the world around her and uses them in arriving at judgments of what she accepts as true.

In professional practice, action is intended to have consequences, and this intention imparts a value component to action. Social work—as work—is intended to achieve change; and this intention is best realized when it is guided by what is the case rather than by what one wishes were the case. To work well, the social worker ought to know; to achieve change, she ought to consider consequences and be guided by values. These assumptions seem essential to an understanding of social work as work that involves significant rational components.

Anticipation

Intent on effecting a process and contributing to the shape of the future, a social worker is constantly anticipating events. Three types of anticipation involving intellectual effort seem essential to our discussion. To be properly understood, the recipient must be related in some way to mental categories previously stored or assigned to a class of recipients with whom he shares some common characteristics. Classification and analogy serve here as modes of anticipation, for they suggest attributes for the specific case that might not be immediately apparent but (because of other evident indicators) appear probable. The worker also anticipates what she will learn about the recipient's past experiences in order to explain how what is came to be. Finally, the worker anticipates the possible consequences of her interventions; and in so doing, she invests the present with the influences of a probable future. These types of anticipation encompass significant intellectual work, involving reasoning of a complex and challenging nature.

Classification and Analogy. Attaching a meaning to attributes of the recipient for the purpose of representation is a necessary aid in identification, and a worker's ability to do this appropriately is one measure of her skill. Each meaning is associated with a class of attributes from which other attributes not previously identified may be inferred. This intellectual work provides the worker with a basis for describing the recipient in a language that communicates to her and to colleagues who use a similar language the form or structure of the service situation. Although classification is necessary, it is not sufficient of itself to develop the meaning of a situation and specify what is important in it. In addition, analogy is essential. Thus, classification and reasoning by analogy are both necessary elements in arriving at an appropriate anticipation of a recipient's manifest condition. The former describes the facts while the latter preserves the form of the relation among them.

In assigning attributes to categories, we are often arranging them in some order that reflects the relationships of classes to one another. The degree to which our knowledge of attributes provides accurate and precise measurements influences our ability to achieve a more or less sophisticated ordering of relationships among classes. Various kinds of ranking, scaling, and propositional statements can define the relationships we believe we find between classes. The sounder our knowledge and the more accurate our descriptions of the phenomena we observe, the more likely that our reasoned anticipations will be fulfilled.

Two characteristics of social work classification appear to influence reasoning in professional work. The process whereby identification and description are achieved, in theory at least, is initiated at the beginning of the professional contact and ends with the termination of service—not before. During the entire service encounter, because there is a potential for new observations, there is also the likelihood of better informed assignment to categories. This potential may not be realized, partly because of psychological influences like the phenomenon of closure and partly because of confusion resulting from an overdose of indigestible data.[3] The process of service nevertheless provides a constant check on classification assumptions and sometimes alters earlier anticipations derived from them. Further, in a specific situation, the attributes used to assign the case to a class diminish in significance as the characteristics that identify the case with a subclass are recognized. In the jargon of the profession, the latter development 'individualizes' each recipient and his situation. When applied to classification in social work practice, a class calculus should be understood in the light of those processes whereby assignments are made to categories.

The integrating character of action for the worker, as she puts together in her own distinctive way what she knows and values, is often discussed but not fully understood.[4] The

3. Martin Wolins, "Selection of Foster Parents: Early Stages in the Development of a Screen" (D.S.W. diss., Columbia University, 1959).

4. C. H. Perelman and Tyteca L. Olbrechts, *The New Rhetoric: A Treatise on Argumentation* (Notre Dame, Indiana: University of Notre

reasoning process whereby this wholeness is achieved in performance is typically analogical. Scott Buchanan's observation of the function of analogy in law and medicine suggests the possibility that this form of reasoning is shared by many professions:

> The whole system of case precedents starts with an initial sort of archetypal case, and the cases are lined up after this. The law grows through analogy. You never get an abstraction out of this. Lawyers don't like to. Of course, it has something to do with the very difficult intellectual process that goes on in a courtroom — making a general law apply to a specific case with all its special circumstances and details. The law is general and as you start the reasoning, you're not sure it's going to apply, but you make it apply through a series of analogies, or precedents. The same thing came up when I was doing philosophy of medicine. This is the way diagnosis works, too. You identify disease through a syndrome of patterns, analogous with each other.[5]

Dame Press, 1969), pp. 371–98; see also Heinz Von Foerster, J.D. White, L.J. Peterson, and J.K. Russell, *Purposive Systems* (London: Spartan Books, 1968); Harley C. Shands, *Thinking and Psychotherapy* (Cambridge: Harvard University Press, 1960); N. Bongard, *Pattern Recognition* (New York: Spartan Books, 1970); Jonathan Burnett, *Rationality* (Atlantic Highlands, New Jersey: Humanities Press, 1969); Frank Barron, "The Psychology of Imagination," *Scientific American* (September 1958); Anthony Wilden, *System and Structure* (London: Tavistock Publications, n.d.), pp. 155–95; George Lukac, *History and Class Consciousness* (Cambridge: MIT Press, 1971), p. xxv: "No purposive activity can be carried out in the absence of an image, however crude, of the practical reality involved"; Glenn Allan Roosevelt, "Metaphoric Understanding," *Social Work* 24, no. 4 (July 1979): 329–30; Robert J. Sternberg, *Intelligence, Information-Processing and Analogical Reasoning: A Componential Analysis of Human Abilities* (New York: John Wiley & Sons, 1977), Chaps. 5, 6; J. R[obert] Oppenheimer, "Analogy in Science," *American Psychologist* 11 (1956): 127–35; R.V. Davis and L.T. Siojo, "Analogical Reasoning: A Review of the Literature," University of Minnesota Department of Psychiatry, Technological Report No. 1 (Minneapolis, 1972); S.E. Whiteley, "Types of Relationships in Reasoning by Analogy" (Ph.D. diss., University of Minnesota, 1973).

5. Harris Wofford, Jr., *Embers of the World: Conversations with Scott*

Social workers rely primarily on compositions of current experiences to initiate storage in memory and recovery from memory of those principles and rules for action associated with previously stored analogous compositions. In practice, the social worker (like the lawyer or doctor) must make her generalized principles and rules apply to specific cases with all their special circumstances and details. She will necessarily use all the tools of reason to achieve this goal. Such tools serve an orienting function and help the worker locate both herself and her client in the unique time and place within which their service roles are enacted, pointing out also the direction in which change ought to move them. The peculiar attribute of analogical reasoning, however, is its capacity for encompassing in one composition the special circumstances and details of the individual case — including much that may be appreciated and understood but not established as known.

Analogy has the virtue and involves the risk of accepting as true much that in fact remains to be established. It allows for a loose association of similar types and frees the worker from a range of uncertainties and doubts that would inhibit action. Reasoning by analogy draws on the worker's imagination, thereby enriching her repertoire of professional activities by capitalizing on the wide range of analogous stored compositions unique to her style and experience. It encourages creativity and originality in practice without forcing her to jettison previously learned principles and rules.[6]

Many risks are entailed in reasoning by analogy. Practice often yields phenomena that look similar but later prove to be essentially different. The attraction of certainty in an action situation may encourage a worker to rely on resem-

Buchanan (Santa Barbara, California: Center for the Study of Democratic Institutions, 1970).

6. Lydia Rapaport, "Creativity in Social Work," *Smith College Studies in Social Work* 38, no. 3 (June 1968): 139–61.

blances between past and present experiences, even in circumstances where the context has changed so radically as to alter the meaning of the same event, even for the same recipient.

As is true of any tool, reasoning by analogy can be used as a crutch to support a weakness in skill that ultimately promotes a dependency that stymies the further development of professional competence. Social work education makes considerable use of social learning procedures. Modeling her practice after that of experienced mentors, a novice may develop a dogmatic adherence to inappropriate analogs justified by faulty theory and therefore acquire a mechanical approach to practice. These risks in the use of reasoning by analogy warn that caution must be exercised in order to avoid its uncritical application. Nevertheless, in situations that require action when unanticipated consequences can be important, choice and decision are necessary, even though the uncertainties inherent in any work intended to shape the future are unavoidable.

The models of practice discussed in social work literature are rarely straightforward replicas of the activities they model. It seems more appropriate to view such models as analogs; and this observation suggests still another caution. Arguments that are validly applied to logical models of formal systems can not be uncritically applied to analogs intended primarily for heuristic purposes in practice.[7]

Social work analogs differ in what they have chosen to model from practice. 'Problem-solving,' which achieved a certain degree of popularity in the last decade, focused on the rational cognitive processes and stressed the applicability of the formal elements of scientific procedures as they appear to operate in the service encounter. The 'helping' model, on the other hand, focused on the roles of the actors and the influence of the setting in the service situation and suggested

7. Mary Hesse, "Models and Analogy in Science," in *Encyclopedia of Philosophy* (New York: Macmillan Co., 1967), 5:354–59.

that the impromptu drama has heuristic value as a replica of practice performance. More recently, systems theory and social-contract theory (among others) have furnished some social workers with models of practice. Whether (for the reason cited or for convenience) we choose to catalogue all nonformal models as analogs or we accept the interchangeable use of these terms common in social work literature, their intended functions are similar: They are expected to provide some meaning and order to the attributes that constitute the basic elements of descriptions and classifications.

The Past. When the worker looks to the past, she is concerned to learn of origins and develop explanations. Although these are not her only concerns, we will consider other uses later. Ideally, the worker is aware of the limits of recall and suspicious of facile assumptions about causality. She looks for facts that meet the criteria of authenticity associated with retrospective inquiries; and she recognizes that knowledge of origins may suggest explanations but not achieve them. For the social worker, explanations are most useful when they both account for all the known facts and suggest others that have not previously been identified.

Explanations in social work must be applicable to a specific case. Thus, explanations about how social injustices have contributed to a recipient's problem condition cannot end with broad generalizations. Evident truths—e.g., the pressures of a slum upbringing; of poverty; of discrimination because of ethnic, racial, or religious origin—must explain how *this* recipient was victimized in his life by *these* social injustices and what *his* response to them did or did not achieve in *his* natural thrust toward health, security, and happiness. In the absence of law-like statements that justify conclusions about specific cases from statistically probable outcomes, the social worker must locate those elements of recipient strength evident in past survival efforts that can be promoted in assisting the recipient to self-realization through his own efforts in the future.[8] This may require—with or without the recipient's full involvement—direct engagement on the part of the worker in efforts to alter the circumstances that she thinks are preserving and perpetuating the injustices that are causally related to the recipient's condition. Such circumstances can often undo and defeat efforts at improvement of this condition through service intervention. The worker seeks etiological explanations through systematic inquiry, utilizing established 'knowns' to summarize her observations and test the hypotheses that give meaning to these observations.

However well developed her knowledge of the etiology of the condition observed, she must establish this specific recipient's unique responses to the factors contributing to his condition. This need is inevitable since the social worker's one pervasive function is to assist the recipient in maximizing his use of service resources, whatever his condition and whatever its origin and causes, expecting that the recipient's efforts (to the degree to which he is capable) will contribute to the achievement of the service objective.

In looking back, the worker may initially seek either to trace the origins of events that link the past to the present or to unravel a stored past recovered from the recipient's recall and corroborated by collateral evidence. In either case, the worker has the option of viewing her own role as that of an observing participant—someone who serves as agent rather than spectator and whose procedures for observing are themselves ingredients in the service relationship. In this view, procedures become important work tools. They have definable impact, they are subject to calculated implementation, and they assist in the accomplishment of a desired end. Accepting the past as currently unalterable but nevertheless influential suggests the variety of uses to which the past may

8. Rudolph H. Weingarten, "Historical Explanation," in ibid., 4:7–12.

be put for service purposes in addition to determining origins and conjectures that explain. In the role of agent, the worker usually has some control over the circumstance under which the past is included in the service encounter. She can influence the scope and character of what will be recovered from memory, when it will be recovered, and how it will be reported. Her capacity to use judgment in choosing from among the possibilities open to her is undoubtedly important in any measure of her competence.

The uses of the past in the present and the uses of classification and analog are directed toward the third type of anticipation, without which practice remains devoid of rational purpose — prediction. In deciding on modes of intervention, the worker must consider their probable outcomes if purpose is to guide her choice of action. In this sense, the future as anticipated consequence enters to shape her work in the present.

Prediction. How does the social worker decide what is to be taken as true or as known? The consequences of action, in our view, includes both past and anticipated outcomes. Any outcomes on which particular truths lay claim for support have resisted violation and remain yet to be exhausted in practice.[9] Although the outcome of a worker's activity may be independent of what has happened in similar circumstances in the past, the past need not be ignored. As a matter of professional practice, moreover, it is unlikely that it would be. Granted that in her daily service activity the worker is most influenced in anticipating consequences by what is occurring in front of her — with *this* recipient under *these* circumstances — and that different workers may perceive these complicated occurrences differently, certain traditional influences act on a worker's understanding of the events she is experiencing. On

9. Nelson Goodman, *Facts, Fiction and Forecast*, 2d ed. (Indianapolis: Bobbs-Merrill Co., 1965), pp. 59–81.

the one hand, the worker will entertain the possibility that certain outcomes cannot be known.[10] This cautions her against an inflexible determinism where human choice acts as an intervening variable. On the other hand, she will rely to some extent on projections from past experiences and on past regularities analogous to mental compositions that arise out of her current experience. Such resemblances confirm previously identified consistencies for her and support their propositional formulations as explanations of observed events and anticipated outcomes.

The worker's view of reality must include the uncertainty that inevitably accompanies her evaluation of the action in which she is involved. This uncertainty may stem from the complexity of the task, from its difficulty, or from its lack of familiarity; and it will be tolerated to the degree that the worker is able to risk action without assurance of possible consequence. Truth and reality in the worker's personal inner-directed perception of her task thus have unusual significance for the work she will perform.

For the social worker, prediction takes on meanings not ordinarily associated with its use as a criterion for asserting the truth of a law-like generalization. The social worker predicts "as much to 'halt' a future as to help it to come into being."[11] The social worker knows that if what has already happened to the recipient determined what will happen to him she would have no reason for intervening in the situation for which her services are sought. Since prediction pertains to what has yet to happen, the worker is as often concerned to prevent an

10. Michael Scriven, "Unpredictability in Human Behavior," in *Scientific Psychology*, ed. Benjamin B. Wolman (New York: Basic Books, 1965), pp. 412–24; Dorothy Emmet, *Rules, Roles and Relatives* (New York: St. Martin's Press, 1966), pp. 109–37.

11. Daniel Bell, "Twelve Modes of Prediction: A Preliminary Sorting of Approaches in the Social Sciences," *Daedalus* 93 (Summer 1968): 873.

undesired occurrence as to promote a desired one. This meaning associated with prediction in practice attaches to practice principles a crucial function in the profession's practice science.

By combining propositional statements and commendations in a single formulation, principles serve as predictive tools to guide action while increasing the range of choices open to the actors. In turn, the activities of both worker and recipient actualize the prediction in work. A principle-determined prediction proposes both what potentially can happen but ought to be avoided and what is possible and should be sought.

The limitations of such principle-sponsored predictions deserve some consideration. If looking back yields no explanation of assorted events for which projections have evolved, it is unlikely that present occurrences will be "consistent" with previously established continuities. Thus one limit on professional predictions is the extent to which the worker has stored relevant analogs. The stronger the claim of the stored retrodiction, the more likely the worker is to accept its predictive value.

Other limitations in professional prediction arise from the complex nature of human behavior in a changing environment. The recipient's experiences range from those of recent origin to others of long and persistent duration. His physiological development is equally variant in time. His understanding and confusion may exist side by side — great wisdom and scholarship next to naiveté and ignorance. Moreover, these very irregular aspects of the recipient and his situation as a unit under observation can combine with even more complex irregular developments within the recipient's environment to warn the worker against any simplistic assumption about what is meant by the phrase "the recipient and his situation." Thus some aspects of a recipient's situation may meet the requisites for predictive formulations more readily than others. Unanticipated consequences may be unequally distributed, thus influencing the worker's effort to evaluate what may happen in the future.

The safest path for the worker is to engage the recipient and hold him to activities that actualize the intended possibilities as they are performed. In effect, this suggests that the greatest certainties associated with professional predictions are likely to be evident in those very areas where the work done actualizes the intended outcomes. Beyond this, anticipated consequences may in fact result from factors over which the worker has little control or influence. This strongly suggests that the effects of social work services at the level of direct intervention are limited by *(1)* a time scale related to the variability of those aspects of the recipient's person and circumstance encompassed in the problem for which he seeks service and *(2)* the direct work done by both worker and recipient on those aspects of the recipient's problem within or closely bound by the period during which they maintain some degree of identifiable service contact. Thus, efforts to describe the work of social workers must tolerate a wide range of measurement imprecision, defined in relation to the nature of both the changes the service is intended to achieve and the decisions such measurements are to support or refute. While seeming to restrict the claim that the profession may make for the consequences of its direct interventions, this suggestion may strengthen the basis on which its 'truths' may be established and its 'realities' affirmed.

Such predictions, however, relate only to the set of outcomes previously described as specific to an individual worker's expectations. They do not include predictions about outcomes of the broader variety that one supposes a community would accept as a basis for sustaining its support of a particular program. The difficulty of attempting predictions of this latter type stems from the influences of complex societal and personal factors on such outcomes—factors beyond the control of the social worker, the recipient, or the agency whose direct services are involved. Often the availability of observation and reporting opportunities, whereby even gross measures of the social scope of problems to be dealt with and the results that can logically be attributed to social work interventions, may be limited. When they are available, they offer unreliable data.

From such a limited perspective, the impact of service on wider social problems would be difficult to determine. Even were we to agree on criterion measures, we have not yet evolved an acceptable and practical procedure for tracing the logical linkage between influences and outcomes. Correlative analyses that might suggest sustained associations require the assumption of a relatively stable community context for practice; but experience suggests caution in assuming such stability, particularly in relation to the conflict-ridden societal problems that are of major concern to social work practice. Earlier we proposed a hypothesis about the limits of professional prediction in the inner-oriented expectation of the worker. At the societal level, prediction in relation to societal criterion variables must likewise be limited by (1) a time scale related to the variability of those aspects of the problem encompassed in the condition for which social services are provided and (2) the work done by workers and recipients on those aspects of the societal problem, within or closely bound by the period during which they maintain some degree of identifiable service contact.

Although the worker anticipates—that is, seeks to describe, explain and predict—in order to qualify her options, she is rarely free in practice to act on all the possibilities she can imagine. Immediate restraints are inherent both in recipient conditions and preferences and in agency policies and procedures. These restraints must be appreciated if purposeful practice encounters are intended.

What Is to Be Worked On? Who Is to Be Worked With?

The matters to be dealt with in the service encounter necessitate formulations that facilitate practice. Whose problems should be dealt with? How should they be defined? What resources are to be allocated to their mitigation? What results are intended? What form are these results to take? These questions inevitably attach themselves to the definition of the professional task.

The unique characteristics of a recipient's situation that assist the worker in individualizing each unit of service have their counterparts in the unique pattern of decisions she makes in arriving at a definition of her role in the provision of service. The worker is aware of both the significant parameters that shape her activities and the need to characterize a particular service encounter within the framework of these parameters.

Thus the worker assumes that in any social service activity the problem to be dealt with can be formulated quite differently by her and the recipient. In order to enter into and sustain a meaningful dialogue with the recipient, she must reconcile this difference. She recognizes that the problems to be worked on carry the imprint of both societal and personal influence. She must appropriately evaluate these influences in each case if her effort is to be directed at significant targets. She knows that both she and the recipient have relevant roles in the service process and that each role has a distinct impact. How control of the process is to be distributed between them is of persistent concern during the service contact. The objectives sought by agency, recipient, worker, and community may be complementary or contradictory. If focus in service is to be maintained, some reconciliation of these objectives is imperative. Finally, it is essential that each encounter be subject to constant surveillance, lest inappropriate and damaging interventions go undetected and helpful ones go unrecognized. The process of evaluation should provide an opportunity for recipient, agency, and community to observe the encounter and to respond with corrective judgments that the worker can weigh in her own evaluations of achievements and failure.

Parameters are sometimes posed as polarities whose interpenetrations and contradictions provide the stimulus for change in the service encounter. In this view, the worker-recipient relationship is characterized by tensions that stem from their differing perceptions and definitions of the problem to be worked on, objectives and control of the process, and appraisal of the service encounter. Where dialogue on these differences can be initiated, service is possible. Where there are no differences, the direct transfer of agency resource to recipient need may be preferable to indirect transfer involving professional social work intervention. When a dialogue is terminated, social work service ends.

As a first step, this discussion suggests no small need for conceptual acumen and an analytical skill on the part of the worker. At every turn, she is driven to arrive at conclusions based on formal, dialectical, and analogical reasoning.

PRIORITIES

THE THREE-FOLD ANTICIPATIONS here described help the worker to characterize each service encounter and prepare her to find her own answers to the priority questions she must inevitably confront in practice. "What should be the order in which I do what I can for this recipient? What should be the order in which we do what we can for this program?" These questions seek a list of possibilities among which a choice must be made, some measure of their interdependence, and the sequence in which those possibilities chosen will be acted on. Thus three different questions are incorporated in one: "What can I do? How does the choice of one influence the other? What order of actions is required?" These three questions differ in the types of answers they seek. The first requests information; the second asks for a propositional statement establishing the relationship of the variables recovered in answer to the first; the third resembles a deliberative question in want of a decision. For each possibility recovered in answer to the first question, a true-or-false test may be applied. In response to the second question, one can propose a procedure for proving whether in fact the relationships specified are what the proposition asserts. The third question calls for a decision rather than an assertion; an answer that is neither true nor false.[12] The first and second questions seek knowledge (i.e., 'truth' statements); the third draws on imperatives. The observation that decisions are predispositions to behave in a certain manner if certain conditions representing tendencies rather than capabilities are realized suggests the value component entailed in an answer to the third question. What the inquirer wants in answer to this question is not a prediction but a suggestion or advice.[13]

A social worker employed by a social agency is not free to exercise her preferences in determining who her recipient will be, what her workload will be, or what problems she will have to deal with. Priority decisions that culminated in the program of services offered by the agency have limited her opportunities. It is not difficult to identify both the prior decisions that have shaped an agency's program and the political and economic interests they reflect. They are implicit in the program budgets of those financing bodies that pass on plans and policy. The agency's goals and objectives, like its policies and procedures, are themselves conditioned by prior decisions; and in turn they set limits within which a worker's choices are exercised.

The worker must deal with two situations that necessitate

12. John M.D. Wheatley, "Deliberative Questions," *Analysis* 15, no. 3 (January 1955): 49–60.
13. Ibid., pp. 52–56.

personal priority decisions, given the constraints that flow from agency program preferences. At any one time, she must decide how to allocate her personal resources among the recipients requiring her services and she must decide on the specific allocation of those resources designated for a particular recipient. I shall not attempt to treat these two decisions separately, although they undoubtedly have distinctive attributes, as well as many in common. Instead, I contrast personal priority decisions with the priority decision process that occurs in social policy and planning activities to highlight their unique attributes.

It is customary in social work to think of priorities as an aspect of the planning and policy decisions of groups, organizations, and communities; but rarely, if ever, is it regarded as an integral part of the worker's practice wherein she decides how to budget and allocate her own personal resources. Actually, the worker's efforts to cope with value preference issues in practice demonstrate all the issues identified in planning and policy choice situations, if we accept the following list of such issues as indicative:

- there are conflicting values at stake;
- value questions must often be posed in "as if" form;
- it is difficult to clarify just what the prevalent values or preferences are;
- there is often dispute as to whose choices are relevant or most relevant to the decisions to be made;
- it is difficult to translate technical issues into their value consequences in a completely objective fashion.[14]

The social worker who works as a planner confronts these issues as an element of her practice function. They are intrin-

14. Alfred J. Kahn, *Theory and Practice of Social Planning* (New York: Russell Sage Foundation, 1969), p. 107.

sic to the service responsibility she is expected to fulfill. In relation to the professional question she puts to herself, however, as she defines her own preferences in the use of her personal resources, her situation does not appear to differ from that of any social worker in direct practice, no matter what area of program interest, problem focus, or interventive process engages her professional talents.

The social worker may accept as a 'given' the agency's allocation of its resources, recognizing the priority choices such allocations reflect in program goals. She may also accept as 'given' the preferences expressed by the recipients of her services about which problems are to be worked on, what is the nature of the help desired, and what outcomes are acceptable. She nevertheless must ask herself, however the restraints of these 'givens' circumscribe her choices, "How shall I allocate my own resources? What investment of self ought I to make in a particular service transaction? In what order should my abilities be committed in meeting the demands visible in this one practice encounter?"

The approaches to decision making suggested for those concerned with problems of valuations in social planning hardly suffice for this inner-directed choice.[15] The former are concerned with processes and procedures for enabling others to achieve consensus on goals and objectives—often in conflict-laden interpersonal situations. Self-directed valuations intended to recover guides for actions that realize the worker's allocation of her own resources involve other matters.

For example, although compromise is often an acceptable ploy in social planning, one does not make compromises *with* oneself, one compromises oneself. Consensus is important to social planners, but one does not look for consensus or majority opinions in inner-choice decisions, nor does one avoid the need to choose by delegating the choice to others—such dele-

15. Ibid., p. 126.

gation is itself the choice. Partializing the circumstances conditioning the need for the self-directed professional priority questions may be helpful, and involving others in identifying alternatives and their consequences may clarify and focus the worker's perspective; but in the end, the worker alone will have to decide how to allocate her resources in each practice encounter within the 'givens' that limit her options.

In this light, the priority decisions of the worker in response to the need condition presented by the recipient and the objective to be achieved by the service, constitute her own 'intake,' specifying her own 'eligibility' and 'ending' criteria.

Social policy and planning efforts to establish a rational procedure for determining priorities have encountered difficulties in four areas:

1. Making qualitatively distinct phenomena quantitatively commensurate;
2. Including the range of interests at stake in the process of priority determination and according them appropriate weight;
3. Assuring channels for altering priorities as circumstances result in undesirable consequences resulting from prevailing priorities;
4. Providing for choices that favor the least advantaged in procedures that reward the advantaged.

These difficulties are believed to be technical in nature; and they are presumed to concern only means. The procedure itself, it is thought, will be largely neutral to the ends it helps to identify. If it were possible to establish that the choice and application of means do not predetermine the scope and range of possible ends to be considered, this presumption would have merit. It seems unlikely, however, that a scheme for determining priorities can be made this neutral to the issues to be considered in its application. For this reason, all phases of the procedure for selecting and ordering goals in policy and planning situations—particularly the 'agenda' that maps what will be considered—are recognized to be influential in determining both choices and the consequences that follow their implementation. In these circumstances, those who benefit most from prevalent distributions of power—political, economic, scientific, and social—will press the technician to take the status quo as a 'given' defining the 'realistic' parameters within which any scheme she proposes should be expected to work. Those who control the resources to be distributed naturally prefer priorities that promise to increase their power, or at least not to weaken their relative positions. Although crisis situations may temporarily loosen their grip on the descision process, it requires a sustained political, economic, scientific, or social upheaval to prevent them from again grasping control of budgeting and allocation. A technician who lacks resources and influence to alter existing power relationships may find it necessary to view 'what is' as the best indicator of 'what is likely to be.' She may be inclined to reject theories and imperatives that basically challenge the existing mode of operation and goal definition, including their order arranged according to preferences. As Aaron Wildavsky concludes,

> In appraising the budgeting process, we must deal with real men in the real world for whom the best they can get is to be preferred to the perfection they cannot achieve. Unwilling or unable to alter the basic features of the political system, they seek to make it work for them in budgeting rather than against them.[16]

What happens to those unable to make the system 'work for them?'

Apparently, theory here justifies methods, and values

16. Aaron Wildavsky, *The Politics of the Budgetary Process* (Boston: Little, Brown & Co., 1964), p. 158.

justify goals, within a prescribed framework assuring their relevance for action. The methods and goals so justified, however, are not neutral to the end result likely to result from the process; in effect, they assure the continuation of present patterns into the future. Certainly, theory and value here fulfill a critical orienting function even as they provide justifications. As noted earlier, the need to act presses the practical man to minimize doubt and maximize certainties. Because 'what is' is taken as a given, in the final analysis this approach to practical problems is conservative. The technician's efforts to make 'what is' work more efficiently may minimize the ill effects that flow from existing inequities; but they seem incapable of overcoming the inequities that produce them.

Do theory and ethics serve a similar justifying function for the worker in relation to her own choices about the use of her personal resources? In some respects they do. For example, in seeking to recover guidelines for action, the worker's theoretical and ethical preferences no doubt point her in certain directions and limit the range of possibilities she will consider in arriving at 'inner' priority decisions. The external parameters that circumscribe her available possibilities (i.e., agency and recipient conditions) certainly restrict her range of choices and serve both a justifying and an orienting function as well. As 'realities' to be reckoned with, they are likely to be accounted for in the theory and ethical preferences of the worker. This tends to assure, whatever the worker's choices, that 'what is' in practice will largely determine 'what should be.' Another element that influences the worker's choice of theory and ethics will be her own response repertoire, which sets limits on what she can personally consider as possible choices.

The worker must also establish a tentative agenda that maps her inner-directed inquiry. This agenda sets forth a set of problems to be dealt with in order that the priority decision appropriately relate to the practical intent of recovery effort. Thus the worker must determine

1. If the recipient has a legitimate claim on her resources;
2. what the recipient would have to do in order to avail himself of these resources;
3. what the worker would have to do to render the agency's services in this instance;
4. what other claims on worker resources are conditioned on this particular allocation, and their relative merit; and
5. what resources are to be allocated in light of the answers to questions 1–4.

The substantive materials that constitute the content that informs these agenda items are generated in the interaction between worker and recipient. Although the worker may be aware of this inner agenda in each service request, she is able to establish the order and scope of her consideration of these items only through exchanges with recipients that occur in the "intake" process itself. Thus, the prevalent view that service begins with the process of determining eligibility and needs no priority decisions seems realistic. It is inevitable that the worker spend a certain amount of her resources determining her time and energy allocations; and this expenditure necessarily influences the direction her relationships with recipients will take. This item apparently ranks first in whatever priority scheme she later decides upon.

The worker's inner-directed agenda must not be confused with the program of work that she and the recipient jointly agree upon to govern their contacts. While the inner agenda is dependent on the outer agenda in certain respects, it is neither temporally nor spatially bound by the latter. The worker's professional questions to herself, while similar to those entering into any priority decision process, nevertheless have unique characteristics that generate their peculiar recovery processes.

The worker's complex self-directed question assumes that there are possibilities (i.e., that a choice exists) and demands that all likely ones be listed. It does not, as far as she is concerned, assume that there is an indeterminate number of such possibilities. The worker seeks answers that commit her existing capacities. Moreover, she has been oriented by agency and recipient conditions, and by her own professional theories and ethics, to remove from consideration all possibilities that do not meet certain special qualifications.

These special qualifications do differ from those that may limit the range of possibilities in social policy and planning. In the first approximation of possibilities, the worker will be guided by "thou shalt nots" that proscribe some cases and focus her attention on recoveries from memory that can count. Such internal censorship obviously cannot prevail in social processes wherein the various interests influencing priority choices must first reach agreement on those shalt nots in order to proceed with the listing of possibilities.

Establishing the interdependence of possibilities in order to arrive at the number of truly independent choices available and determining which choices necessitate others as prerequisites or consequences can only follow, not precede, the listing of possibilities. This sequence, of course, is not unlike the one evident in the interplay of preferences in interpersonal and intergroup priority processes. In the self-directed query, however, both the possibilities and their associations are presumed to be likely and to be in the interest of the recipient. In social policy and planning choices, this is hardly the case when heterogenous interests are represented.

In any case, the initial priority decision cannot precede some approximation of responses to the questions noted at the outset of this discussion. Nor is the worker committed to an unbreakable chain of consequences in arriving at her initial decision. It is not probable that all possibilities and their interdependences will be recovered or discovered in time for the initiation of action. The process is continuous and feedback opens new options not previously stored. In addition, stored options are sometimes recognized as appropriate only after the worker–recipient interaction develops.

In the social planning situation, collective decisions are usually reached only after a considerable investment of effort on the part of those whose interests are represented. These decisions are not easily altered, and they are not as susceptible to change in the course of their implementation through the corrective influence of feedback. Resources committed to one purpose often deny sustenance to others, thus terminating the representation of certain interests in policy and planning decision-making bodies and denying them further claim to a voice in setting or altering priorities.

The decision made in response to a self-directed question may more readily be altered as a result of experience during its implementation. Because the commitment it entails is private, it is more open to self-correction — not having to contend with the fault-finding that publicly admitted error in political judgments normally provokes. Although the worker's resources are limited and allocations to one purpose will deplete resources to be used otherwise, to the degreee that the decision is the product of a single judge, judgments will be contingent on self-selected criteria that reflect the worker's natural preference for flexibility in investing herself in a practice engagement.

A unique aspect of the self-directed professional question is its monostylous nature. What the worker finds attractive will more than likely influence her preferences. Since the alternatives to be ordered are inseparable from the style in which they are formed, the elements of style conflict or style complementarity one finds in interpersonal decisions are absent from the worker's inner choices. Stylistic bent affects inner-directed query in another unique fashion.[17] The worker expects that she will have to carry out in practice whatever she decides. Knowing this, she is likely to prefer those alternatives she judges most congenial to her own style. Thus style influences the alternatives selected for consideration and affects their ranking. For this reason, it is not surprising to observe how often diverse situations requiring dissimilar activities on the part of the worker nevertheless manifest her individual style in their realization.

We have deliberately contrasted social priority determination with personal, hoping to use their differences to clarify elements peculiar to the inner-directed priority query. The comparison was also intended to highlight similarities that suggest the political attributes of professional thought processes. This subject deserves more discussion than it has been given. Nevertheless, it seemed important to identify it, since a worker's priority decisions inevitably influence her practice; but they are rarely recognized for what they are: her own approximation of her view of just and trustworthy behavior.

If we accept the merit of this discussion of the priority question, the importance of stored information, rules, and principles becomes clear. If recovery is to be efficient and appropriate, it will have to respond to the three types of questions incorporated into the one priority question. Ideally, fixed priority schedules, already established and stored and readily recoverable, would effectively meet this requirement. Such schedules enter the worker's memory during her educational preparation and her own practice. Priority rules and principles thus become part of her professional knowledge and thus can be recovered in a manner not unlike that assumed for other rules and principles. In situations not com-

17. T. A. Sebeok, *Style in Language* (Cambridge: MIT Press, 1960), pp. 289–92.

posable into professional questions — those for which stored analogs do not exist — the three types of answers must be recovered in the sequence described earlier. Fortunately, these situations will be infrequent in a practice largely governed by rules; they will be more frequent where appeals to principles are common; and they will characterize a practice in which principles and rules have yet to develop. In the last instance, the decision process will be prolonged and action will be inhibited.

There is no model that purports to describe the manner in which an individual manages to arrange inner-determined possibilities in priority order. There is much material dealing with this aspect of priority determination as it occurs in the social policy and planning area, particularly in relation to budgetary processes. These descriptions, however, generally assume parameters missing from the inner decision process and omit some we know to be present. Rather than hypothesize what the inner process may involve, I should like to note only this important omission in this discussion.

The nature of the reasoning entailed in a professional practice and the complexity of the reasoned responses a worker must make to priority questions has hardly been fully explored in this brief introduction. Nevertheless, it should be evident from this discussion why the reasoning part of professional action is its most important component.

Perspective

If this discussion of the reasoning process has provided some insight into the underpinnings of the intellectual work of a professional practice, it has done so at some sacrifice of perspective. The work and the worker are strongly influenced by the time and place, by the history and culture that provide the context of practice. It would be a serious omission to conclude this analysis without even a brief effort to locate the work and the worker in the wider social context. The final chapter considers some salient aspects of the influence of context on practice.

CHAPTER THIRTEEN

»»   ««

Context

I HAVE USED the work paradigm as an aid in the analysis of the cognitive elements of professional practice. I hope this paradigm has helped the reader to maintain a consistent appreciation of the relationships among these elements. The concept of work was also intended to remind the reader that professional practice, while essentially intellectual, is nevertheless work. As an introductory effort, the analysis stopped far short of a full treatment of the complexities involved in the mental work described. Although the discussion is sensitive to the historical, cross-cultural, and generative aspects of such work, these influences were not directly addressed. Rather, the somewhat static and abstract nature of the paradigm served to introduce essential building blocks with which a more ambitious analysis can be pursued. Nevertheless, granted the limited scope of what has been attempted, mention should be made of certain pervasive contextual influences that locate these building blocks in time and space.

It is unlikely that there will be full agreement among professional social workers on means for achieving their goals and on the ends to be sought by professional effort. Social workers are employed in a variety of fields; in diverse communities; and in social milieus that include a full spectrum of culture, class, race, ethnic, age, and sex differences. Their perspectives are inevitably influenced by the peculiarities of their practice context, which in turn affect their choice of practice principles.

Social workers assume ideological positions in their choice of practice principles. These choices, however, are not unaffected by the preferences of the community at large and by the recipients of service. These societal pressures are filtered in turn through organizational priorities that contribute to choices affecting workers' decisions. Because social workers occupy a range of positions in organizational hierarchies from executive director to line worker, while some are individual entrepreneurs operating outside the constraints of organizational policies, these influences are complicated still further. Workers' economic and political interests are necessarily responsive to the positions they occupy. Choices of practice principles encapsulate all these influences and shape the worker's ideology.

The intellectual tools employed by social workers are not theirs exclusively. They are utilized in the skillful practice of all professions. In limiting the analysis to one profession, I have not considered the differences that characterize the uses of these tools in other professions but are implicit in the examples drawn exclusively from social work.

In their form and structure, tools convey the accumulated wisdom of the past that contributed to their power and relevance. Intellectual tools are no exceptions. They too are subject to refinement, prone to obsolescence, and likely to become dysfunctional as experience and practice set new tasks to be accomplished. While they are not *things* in the ordinary view of tools as marketable commodities, they too can be stored and recalled at will.

Their use value may persist over time. When it is not employed in practice, however, the power of these intellectual tools can dissipate. Thus the worker who wishes to be skillful in their use must invest time and effort to keeping them fresh in mind and attuned to changing circumstances. Although the analysis did not directly consider how these attributes of the intellectual aids to practice are managed by the profession, it did appreciate that this management is of some significance. Social workers are mobile professionals in a highly fluid labor market. Many practitioners experience periodic interruptions in their work histories—including lengthy withdrawals from practice for personal and practical reasons. When they seek to update their skills in order to reenter the profession or prepare for a change in field or modality of practice, the building blocks considered in this text may prove helpful in guiding their retooling efforts.

Finally, the analysis did not directly address the status of social workers within the wider class structure of society. Although some are self-employed in profitable private practice and others are salaried managers of enterprises, the overwhelming majority are salaried employees of organizations that they neither own nor govern. When we refer to them as workers, it is hardly appropriate to assign the same status to them that we would attribute to workers in industry or commerce. In many respects, social workers are a middle class, with ideologies not unlike those of other professionals who depend on their own labor rather than that of others for a livelihood. An analysis of the influence of their class position on their preferences would also move the discussion from an introductory level to a more sophisticated level.

These and similar but broader contextual issues, although they were not directly addressed, were not ignored in the analysis of social work as work. An effort has been made throughout to present the fundamentals so as to assure their consistency with the broader and deeper understanding of the work involved that a more sophisticated analysis would achieve.

I have assumed that in the long run one can expect the work of social workers to undergo major changes as the context of practice changes. It is likely, however, that the structure of the mental work described in this book will change far less and at a slower rate than the substantive content on which these tools for thought will be employed.

Index

>>»   ««<

A

Ability, 57
Accountability, 20, 45, 183
Action, 41, 50, 57, 59, 64, 84, 105, 107,
    111, 130, 133, 147, 162, 166–168,
    170, 179, 190, 197, 213, 223–224,
    228, 233, 247, 249
  Discriminatory, 84
  Imposed (Inhibited), 65
  Punitive, 84
  Prescribed, 152
  Suspended, 65
Advanced professional (Expert). *See* Skill,
    dimensions of
Agency, 77, 131–132, 181, 199, 208,
    237–238
  Induction of, 20–30
Agency resources, 143, 199. *See also*
    Variables, independent
Alternate frames of reference, 80
Alternatives, 48, 58, 65
  Theoretical formulations of, 173
Analogs, 76, 196, 203, 229–230
  Conceptual, 65, 66, 74–75
Analogy, 225–226, 228. *See also*
    Reasoning by analogy
Ancillary information, 166
Anticipation, 224–225
Application, 55
Approach, problem-solving, 116–117
Aptekar, Herbert, 191
Assessment, 15, 130, 167, 194, 198, 202
Association, 65, 163
Assumptions, 224
Awareness, 126, 152
  Focal, 152
  Subsidiary, 152
Unconscious, 70

B

Behavior, 20, 37, 50, 129, 132, 136,
    151–153, 163–165, 170, 179, 197,
    204, 210, 217, 223, 234, 248
  Ethical, 183
  Habituated, 163
  Predictable, 163
  Systematic, 163
Behavioral norms, 133, 137
Belief, 49, 108–109, 127, 129, 133,
    135–138, 204
Buchanan, Scott, 227

C

Certainties, 70
Change, 9–10, 41–42, 53, 62–63, 100,
    114
  Inner-directed, 211
  Objective measurement of, 37
  Potential, 37
Checklist syndrome, 167
Choices, 13, 55, 57–58, 64–65, 73–74, 86,
    88, 95–96, 112–113, 127–132, 141,
    144, 164–165, 172, 192–193,
    197–198, 202–203, 208–211,
    213–214, 224, 229, 234, 238–244,
    246, 248, 251
  Inner-directed, 241
  Value, 71
Commands, 42, 49, 51–53, 81, 88, 90,
    127–128, 133, 136, 139, 143, 169,
    173, 196
  Prescriptive, 83
Commendations, 12, 42, 56, 81, 90, 101,
    128, 133–135, 137–139, 143–144,
    183
Commission, 62

INDEX

Community, 181, 183–184, 201, 208, 215, 237–238, 251
  Expectations, 204–205, 213
  Norms, 181, 205, 209–210
Component, 169
Compenent Value, 169
Composition, 69
Condition, 180, 182, 225, 239
Condition to be altered, 9–11, 13, 30–32, 34, 37, 41, 73, 148, 177, 180, 185, 194, 204
Confidentiality, 43–44
Conflict, 102, 136, 144–145, 182
Consequences, 27, 29, 130, 134, 192, 197, 199, 201, 216, 219, 225, 229, 232–233, 235, 240, 242–243, 247
Context, 251–253
Control, 42, 156, 179–180, 199, 219
Credibility, 27

D

Decisions, 48, 73, 125, 141, 166, 168, 182, 191–192, 194, 229, 235, 237, 239–241, 244, 246–249, 252
Decisions of practice, 127
Decisions of principle, 131
Determinism, 95, 233
Direction, 42, 49
Directives, 42–45, 50–53, 55, 68–69, 71, 74, 80, 127, 133, 143–144, 169–170, 173, 192
Discovery, 66
Discrimination, 102
Doubts, 70, 193

E

Effect, 36
Effort, 253
  Intellectual, 164
  Misdirected, 11
  Professional, 251
  Recovery, 65
Environment, 18, 67
Equality, 86–87, 93, 97
Equity, 86–87, 92–93, 199
Ethical conviction, 127
Ethical dilemma, 57

Ethical imperatives, 42, 58, 65, 83, 87, 90, 92, 96, 98–99, 101, 128, 133, 137–139, 141, 145, 168, 170, 173, 183
Ethical prescriptions, 170
Ethics, 12, 19, 71, 105, 118, 127, 138, 220, 244, 246
  Code of, 83, 89, 94, 131, 138, 142
  Professional, 132
Evaluation, 178
Evidence, 178, 198
  Adequacy of, 109
  Empirical, 203
  Observable, 126
Exchange, internal, 68
  Oral, 68
Exchange value, 36. *See also* Value
Expectations, 169, 197
Experience, 21–22, 52, 63, 103, 113, 202, 217, 233
Explanations, 75, 230

F

Factors, 180
Faith, 115–117, 138, 163
Fate, 163
Freedom, 148
Function, 113, 178, 190, 207, 214–217, 219, 228, 230, 234, 244
Functional approach, 207–212, 218–220
Functional formulation, 211
Functional practice, 208, 212, 240
Functional school, 207
Functional social work, 76, 80, 213
Function theory, 193

G

Generalizations, 75, 78, 95, 157, 233
"Givens," 132–133, 213–214, 241–243
Global terms, 155–156. *See also* Style, global
Goals, 11, 13, 25, 30, 32–33, 49, 51–52, 55–56, 67, 71, 99, 114, 127, 131, 137, 139, 142, 144, 169, 182, 184–185, 196–201, 214, 216–217, 228, 239, 241, 243–244, 251
  Actual, 181
  Ideal, 181

Goals of social work, 199, 202–207

H

Habitual response, 136
Habituation, 70
Hall, Edward, 154, 158
Helping situations, 64
Hypotheses, 80, 137, 154, 163, 203, 231, 236, 249

I

"If-then" propositions. *See* Proposition, process
Imagination, 170
Imperatives, 71, 131–134, 138, 142–143, 243
Indeterminate situation, 64
Induction, 91
Inequity, 170, 244
Inference, 74
Informed judgments, 127
Inner-choice decisions, 241
Inner-directed inquiry process, 203
Inner-directed questions, 68. *See also* Professional question
Insight, 163
Intellectual efforts, 15
  Discovery and invention, 15
  Experiment and demonstration, 15
  Trail and error, 15
Intention, 36, 53, 55, 57, 88, 95, 128, 133, 136, 142, 153, 168–170, 192
Internal interrogatory process, 69
Intervention, 15, 33, 51, 88, 189–221, 225, 231–232, 235–236, 238
Intuition, 163
Investment of effort, 10
Issues, cognitive, 172
  Ethical, 172

J

Judgments, 11, 19, 24, 27, 36, 50, 52, 62–63, 73, 108, 110, 125, 127–128, 131, 133, 136–137, 144, 157, 161, 164, 166, 169, 171, 179–180, 183, 185, 196–197, 206, 223–224, 232, 238, 247

Judgments *(continued)*
  Personal, 163
  Professional, 167
Justification, 53, 58, 169, 173, 201, 208, 244

K

Knowledge, 49, 57, 64–66, 76, 86, 99, 111–112, 116, 126, 134–135, 138, 140, 144, 161–162, 171, 181, 185, 190, 195–197, 206, 210, 212–213, 215, 220, 225–226, 230–231, 239, 248
  Empirical, 107
  Personal, 107, 120–126

L

Levels of intellectual demand, 164
Logic, 36

M

Memory, 63–64, 147, 228
Method, 162, 167–168, 244
Models, 138, 190, 203, 211, 229–230, 249
  Nontheoretical, 76
  Theoretical, 76. *See also* Theory, relevant
Models of behavior, 137–138
Models of practice, 76
Moral perspectives 133
Mores, 184
Motivation, 18, 141

N

Needs, 11, 13, 15, 32–33, 36, 67, 78, 103, 134, 177, 181–182, 186–187, 205–206, 208–209, 212–213, 218–219, 223, 231, 242
Norms, 141, 143–145, 205, 210
  Agency, 142, 144
  Operational, 142

O

Objectives, 11, 13, 25, 32–33, 55, 71, 182–184, 196, 200, 204, 231, 237–239, 241

INDEX

Obligations, 22
Observations, 50, 67, 180, 236, 239
Omission, 62, 179, 249
Options, 144–145, 166, 231, 236, 242, 247
Options for action, 165
Outcome, 203–205, 236, 241
Outcome measures. *See* Variables, dependent

P

Participants. *See* Relationship, worker-recepient
Performance, 80
Perspective, 249–250
Poincaré, 154
Positioning Statements, 73
Practice, 41–59, 63, 67–68, 105, 125, 129, 133, 135, 151, 198, 226, 228, 234, 248
Practice principle, 42–44, 56–57, 62–63, 87, 89–90, 102, 118, 133, 144, 170, 207, 234, 252
Practice theory, 63, 76, 193
Prediction, 232, 234–235
Preprofessional (Technician), *See* Skill, dimensions of
Principles, 41–42, 51, 54, 65–66, 100, 105, 127, 136, 139, 148, 205, 212, 216, 228, 249
Principles of process, 214
Principle-seeking question, 57
Priorities, 238–249
Procedures, 183. *See also* Method
Process, 56, 66–67, 210, 216–221, 223, 226, 237–238, 247
Professional practice, 147, 150, 159, 192, 196, 202, 223–224, 232, 249–250
Professional preference, 198
Professional questions, 65–67, 71, 73
Professionals, 16–17, 19, 21, 29–30, 41–42. *See also* Skill, dimensions of
Propositional assumptions, 134
Propositional statements, 194
Propositions, 42, 62, 127, 144, 163–165
  Causal, 62, 74
  Explanatory, 138
  Process, 62, 74, 169
  Theory-based, 173

Purpose, 11, 22, 41–42, 48, 56, 127, 181, 183, 214, 223
  Definition of, 12

R

Rawls, John, 98
Reasoning, 37, 86, 111
Reasoning by analogy, 58, 74, 225, 228–229
Recall, 65, 67
Recipients, 16–17, 20, 22, 27, 30–37, 64, 76, 89, 93, 97, 116, 129, 132, 169, 206, 208–209, 214, 217, 225, 229–230, 235, 237, 240, 245
Recovery, 50, 66, 206, 248
  Definition of, 12
Relationships, 62, 198
  "If-then" and "from this in time to that," 62
  Worker-recipient, 218
Resources, 33–35, 52, 78, 141, 145, 170, 180, 184–185, 209, 211, 217, 231, 240–241, 243, 245
Responses, 168
Responsible, 44–45, 47, 51, 62, 128, 214, 218
Richmond, Mary, 194
Risk, 156, 228–229
Roles, 180, 190, 206–209, 217, 219–220, 231, 237
Rules, 41–44, 47–51, 53–54, 57, 66, 105, 118, 120, 127, 134–135, 143–144, 148, 163–164, 169, 193, 196, 203, 205, 228, 248–249
  Characteristics of, 49
Rule-seeking questions, 57

S

Sanctions, moral, 145
Self-awareness, 37, 120, 193
Self-determination, 133
Self-directed question, 68–69, 247
Self-directed valuations, 241
Self-evaluation, 28
Self-fulfillment, 130, 132
Sense impressions, 67

INDEX

Service, 15–16, 18–19, 30, 46, 48, 55, 67, 78, 93, 119, 129, 138, 169, 177, 181, 185–187, 207, 209, 211, 215, 226, 235, 237–238, 240–241, 252
Setting. *See* Agency
Signals, 74
Simon, Herbert A., 79
Skill, 20, 119, 144, 159, 161–173, 177, 184–185, 187, 195, 199, 202, 213, 223, 229, 238, 253
  Degrees of, 163
  Dimensions of, 173
Smalley, Ruth, 195
Social contract theory, 98
Social justice, 141
Social work, 23, 30, 34–37, 41, 44, 55, 59, 75, 80, 108, 129, 139, 142, 159, 197, 206, 219, 221, 252–253
Social workers, 16, 43, 63, 75, 130–132, 142, 202, 212, 239, 253
  Attributes of, 17–18
Societal conditions, 140
Standards, 44
Strategies, 189–190
Style, 67, 113, 120, 147–148, 150–156, 159, 171–172, 185, 247–248
  Analytic, 156
  Global, 156
  Idiosyncratic, 156
  Individual, 152–153
  Institutional, 152
  Personal, 152–153, 155
  Urban, 155

T

Tactics, 189, 190
Taft, Jessie, 158–159
Tasks, 44, 53–54, 56, 58, 114, 117, 151, 164–165, 168, 171, 190, 221, 224, 233, 252
  Professional, 237
Technique, 41, 166
Theory, 18, 61–63, 66, 71, 105, 127, 138, 163–164, 181, 220, 243–244, 246
  relevant, 65
Theory of practice, 147

Time, 24, 45, 55, 57, 65, 157, 159, 182, 216, 235, 245, 249
Titmuss, Richard, 140
Trust, 94, 102
Truth, 25, 55, 70, 91, 105, 109–110, 132, 137, 140, 144, 163, 191, 233, 235
  Evident, 230
Truth Statements, 128

U

Use value, 36, 107, 252. *See also* Values

V

Values, 13, 19, 21, 24–25, 28–29, 42, 57, 64, 66, 84–85, 90, 105, 127–129, 131, 134–135, 139–140, 142, 145, 161–162, 170, 198, 205–206, 210, 220, 224, 230, 240, 243–244:
  Definition of, 12
  Dominant, 134
  Fundamental, 169
Value Judgments, 127–133
  Definition of, 128
Variables, 202–204, 239
  Dependent, 55
  Independent, 55
Verification, 137

W

Wildavsky, Aaron, 243
Will. *See* Intention
Work, 11, 15, 30, 43–45, 48, 53, 59, 85, 118, 141, 144, 147, 153, 161, 249–251, 253
  Concept of, 9 10
  Elements of, 9–10, 59, 061, 177–187
  Intellectual, 9–10, 63, 164, 223, 225, 249
  Manual, 9–10
  Theoretical, 63
Work units. *See* Tasks
Workers, 43, 47–50, 52–54, 56–57, 61, 64, 68, 77, 105, 127–128, 144–145, 182, 209–210, 216–217, 219, 223–224, 233, 237, 245, 248–250